Pranayama *Yoga* for Health and *Happiness*

HIMADRI LAHIRY

AuthorHouse™ UK
1663 Liberty Drive
Bloomington, IN 47403 USA
www.authorhouse.co.uk
UK TFN: 0800 0148641 (Toll Free inside the UK)
UK Local: 02036 956322 (+44 20 3695 6322 from outside the UK)

This book is printed on acid-free paper.

ISBN: 979-8-8230-8829-9 (sc)
ISBN: 979-8-8230-8830-5 (e)

Library of Congress Control Number: 2024912146

Print information available on the last page.

Published by AuthorHouse 06/18/2024

authorHOUSE®

Pranayama *Yoga* for Health and *Happiness*

What is beyond the cosmos?
Let us discover.....

PREFACE

In preparing this book the main aim has been to retain the basic message of Pranayama yoga while omitting practices that are obviously not suitable for everybody. There are many advantages of learning and practicing Pranayama yoga. These practices and exercises have been purposely emphasised. Basically the word Pranayama is the technique of breathing where Prana means the vital energy or life force and Yama means the extension or expansion of the life force by controlling the timing of our breathing, inhaling, retaining and exhaling which provides oxygenated blood to our entire body and its organs.

It has been written with a view to give the correct and comprehensive and scientific information on all the different aspects of Pranayama to discern between the essential and the optional parts of the different techniques of Pranayama.

The Second chapter of this book discusses the philosophy and history of pranayama yoga and explains the concept and application of Prana, the sum total energy of the universe. It explains the concept of pranayama as seen in yogic literature, how it developed and how so many techniques of pranayama came into existence.

Chapter three deals with simply the preliminaries of Pranayama yoga.

Chapter four explains a brief view of scientific research and analysis of Pranayama studied by several eminent scientists by referring to the functions and benefits of our internal systems of the body such as: circulatory system, respiratory system, endocrine system, digestive system, nervous system and the effects on mental hygiene. It also deals with how to practice for proper functioning of our body.

Chapter five explains in details the breathing techniques of Pranayama, concept of Nadi (subtle channels through which energy of Prana flows) of the Chakras (the concentrated energy centers of the body) incorporating and emanating energy to keep us functioning at optimal levels and also explains how to practice the breathing exercises and their benefits.

Chapter six explains the method of Kumbhaka, (retention of the breathing techniques) of Pranayama.

Chapter seven, deals with general advice and preparing for the pranayama exercises such as worming up and cooling down methods of our body with explicit diagrams together with precaution before practicing.

Chapter eight, deals with different types of Pranayama and their benefits.

Chapter nine explains different Mudras (hand gestures) and their benefits used while practicing Pranayama.

In Chapter ten, some of the cooling down exercises have been explained.

At various places in this book the original source from where the particular point under discussion is picked up, is indicated by a reference. An attempt has been made to present many concepts in as much a precise and clear- cut manner as is possible. It certainly establishes that Pranayama is one of the most potent and effective techniques which influence our body and mind in a remarkable way.

There are many 'quick fix' cosmetic aids for mental as well as physical benefits and of self-improvement available today such as weight loss supplement, cosmetic surgery and other health products and methods. Of all such available aids that are available today, yoga is certainly the most reliable, safest and the best because of its natural methods and techniques and without any side effects.

The author, Professor Lahiry's yoga classes in Singapore, UAE, Turkey and England, many dramatic positive changes have been seen in several students practising yoga there. Some of these transformations are slow and gradual; however, others are quite fast and dramatic. People of all ages have reported that yoga has positively helped them to increase enjoyment and enrichment of their lives.

Although yoga is widely used to improve the physical health by improving muscle tone and reducing weight etc. another most remarkable feature of yoga is its ability to change a person's attitude and in turn providing a more serene outlook to their appearance and activities. Practicing yoga for some time has certainly changed their attitude towards mental development as they have learnt to relax even at a very disturbed situation by toning up their muscles, glands and whole of the internal system.

For improving and enriching the life, needs simple instruction, guidance and encouragement. The author has attempted to instil such interest in this book. Behind the writing of this book comes more than forty five years of experience of teaching and research including (along with many others) the field of yoga. After completing his yoga training in India and then becoming a British Citizen. Prof.Lahiry has taught Yoga and Pranayama to hundreds of students and has had ample opportunity to observe theirr positive effects.

This book mainly emphasises and simplifies the physiological benefits of Pranayama yoga (breathing exercises). As far as possible, the author has explained with scientific validation so that the readers can understand, can apply and choose the exercises they need for their own purpose. It is also assumed that before practicing Pranayama, you have learnt and have been practicing some of the important yoga Asana which are necessary and complements Pranayama. There are sections in this book explained in details the ways of preparing for exercises; the warming up and cooling down processes; and breathing exercises of Pranayama. Clear drawings and diagrams are given as and when required to illustrate exercises and where appropriate.

Pranayama can be practiced by both male and female. The female figures in this book are deliberately drawn to emphasise the intended idea to instil in this book.

These notes about Pranayama are strictly based upon the synthesis, vital, operative and research conclusions on the ancient yoga texts and traditions, besides being presented in the light of modern sciences and are thus meant to serve as a reliable practical guides to the earnest students of Pranayama yoga.

The author wishes to emphasise that even though this book has been written in a simplified manner for the readers to practice at home, as far as practicable, 'Pranayama' should be learnt from a qualified and experienced teacher at least in the initial stage of learning. The simplified scientific explanation will certainly help readers in the absence of teacher to their advantage, however, it is advised, and before embarking on the practice of Pranayama yoga, the readers must take medical approval to ensure that nothing forbids them to practice certain exercises. It is also advised to follow the instructions carefully as mentioned in the book.

December, 2019   Prof. Himadri Lahiry

Wolverhampton, U.K.

Contents

LIST OF DIAGRAMMES

CHAPTER ONE

Introduction

It has been suggested by many professionals and in Indian scriptures-Vedas, that there are three path of development of the self, which are the physical side, the mental side and the spiritual side. The whole purpose of practicing yoga is to enhance these areas of a person. There are several paths of yoga those coincide with all of these three aspects of the self. For example, the yoga for wisdom, the yoga for knowledge, the yoga for higher faculties, and the yoga for devotion, which are concerned with enhancing the physical side of the self, the mental side of the self and the spiritual side of the self. If people can enhance all these areas themselves at the very highest possible point, it can bring many advantages to the person. All these paths of yoga, begins with Hatha yoga, the oldest existing physical-culture system in the world, followed by the next important part of the yoga, which is both the mental & physical side of the yoga, is "Pranayama".

The word 'Hatha'in Sanskrit is made up of the syllable ha, meaning 'moon' and tha, which means the 'sun'. According to yogis there are two warring impulses those are set in motion in our body every time we breathe. The 'moon' impulse is called 'prana vayu' that begins in the heart and ascends to the brain. Whereas the 'sun impulse which is called 'apana vayu' starts at the solar plexus and heads downwards to the anus. The imbalance and the discord between these contrary pulls cause the restlessness of the mind we experience in our body. The breathing exercises (Pranayama) are designed to create the uniting of these two currents.

'What then happens is that the concentration of energy is pushed down to the base of the spine. Here according to yogis is situated one of the seven chakras (the energy centres) of the body and the Susumna, (the central spinal canal)'

Pranayama is a part of the path of mental concentration and also the 'health-care'. It covers a broad area of human life. Health-care encompasses the life as a whole covering its physical, mental, social and environmental aspects. Pranayama is basically the art of controlling breath.

It is the method of breathing exercises within the large science of yoga. Although to interpret Pranayama as 'breathing exercises' would be to limit sadly the scope of the exercises and to misunderstand their true purpose. It is a process of collecting, storing and making conscious control of the vital Pranic energies in our bodies.

Pranayama is derived from the root word "Prana"(mysterious occult life force), the sum total of all the energy of the universe which consist of the sky (Akasa), the cosmic ether. "Yama", is a disciplined method and control of Prana, the life giving vital force to curb or to master. The science of controlling Prana is "Pranayama".

The aim of pranayama is to increase the absorption and fixation of Prana to accumulate in specific centre and distribute this energy throughout the body. To understand the methods of Pranayama, the history and philosophy of Pranayama must be studied. The history part shows its gradual emergence and development while philosophy establishes its basic principles, revealing its fundamental strength as a discipline. If the philosophy is correct, the discipline is sure to survive, otherwise in course of time a stronger doctrine might wipe it off.

In preparing this book, the main aim has been to retain and explain the basic rules, techniques, practice methods at different stages of Pranayama with scientific explanation, while omitting many practices of asana of Hatha yoga. However, some asana which are important for practicing Pranayama have been included.

Philosophically, as per explanation of Indian scriptures it says that there are in living bodies all around us such as Akasa (sky), contains mainly the best and most benign principles (Sattva) which is responsible for sound, the sense of hearing, and functional subdivisions of the blood vessels and sinews (that which joins a muscle to bone) into minute capillaries etc. According to Samkhya branch of philosophy, "Vayu (air) comprises of most active principle, (Rajas) mainly accounts for physical and physiological activities of Pranayama". However, when we discuss body and its perfect development by practicing yoga and Pranayama we must accept that the body undergoes certain changes at certain stages which are normal and inevitable. The childhood, the adolescence or puberty, the youth and the old age are the different stages in persons' look and behaviour accordingly. The essence of Pranayama yoga is to optimise the Pranic energies in our bodies at various stages of life.

Every effort has been made to trace all copyright holders but, if any have been inadvertently overlooked, the author will gladly receive information enabling him to rectify any effort or omission in subsequent editions.

This book brings a fresh approach to the practice of Pranayama, and emphasis is on understanding the principles as well as practical application based on Indian scriptures in scientific validation and provides a comprehensive and logically arranged scheme of Pranayama practice.

It is a pleasure for me to record my sincere appreciation to my family. My children- Susmita, Suvadri and Soma- have been an encouragement and inspiration in producing the book. My share of labour involved in producing this book was greatly reduced by Mrs. Manjusha Lahiry, my wife, and I thank her for her patient and invaluable assistance.

I have great faith and hope that readers will benefit from the information and knowledge contained in this publication.

Written By:

Prof. Capt. Himadri Lahiry
B.Sc (L'Pool), M.A., M.B.A. (Stirling), Master Mariner (F.G.)
Cert Ed, (Lancs), F.E.E Ats Academy (USSR), B.Mus. (India),
MNI, MRIN, MI MarTech, FRMetS.
Life member of The National Cultural Association (India)
Life member of Sanskrit Natya Parishad. Vidya Vachaspati,(Ajmer Shastra Pith).

CHAPTER TWO

Philosophy and History of Pranayama Yoga

Philosophy is the basic and also structural frame of any discipline. Without philosophy it cannot develop rationally. Reasoning faculties, logistics and an effort to explain away the obstinate loopholes are the special features of philosophy. Life without philosophy, in whatever shape it might be, cannot sustain. Pranayama in yogic discipline had to have a philosophy to develop and survive so many years with positive outcomes. Every living being is described by the Indian philosophical systems as an individual (karmapurusa) in union with mind, sense organs and material body. The human body and its functions are always a matter of mystery. Anatomy is the science of most form and structure of organic bodies. Our body acts and reacts automatically all the time. Proper body functioning is synonymous with healthiness. Any disorder caused by emotional or external condition leads to abnormal body functions. According to Indian philosophy, "seat of consciousness, composed of the aggregate of the products of five mahabhutas (fundamental matters) viz: earth, water, fire, air, space and carrying on in the state of equilibrium and body components according to division in smallest units (cells) are innumerable, due to over-abundance, over-minuteness and transcending perception. The causative agent in conjunction and dis-conjunction of cells is Vayu (air) and also the nature of activities" According to modern physiology, the frontal lobe of the human brain is the centre of all mental faculties i.e. intellect, knowledge, memory, talent etc. The other centres of the brain have close connections and cooperation with this centre. In post-mortem examination, of idiotic, paralytic and insane persons' frontal lobe of the brain were found either underdeveloped or damaged. It has also been tested that the centre of thinking, debating, taking proper judgement, rationalisation and determination, although placed differently in the brain, work in unison when necessary as a coordinator. If somehow the mind remains inoperative, all these organs cannot perform. The Pranayama exercises to apply and use 'Prana' will help to understand the advantages in a person's life.

According to Swami Sivananda, "Prana is the sum total of all the energy in the universe. This is surely something vast. For the yogis, the universe is composed of Akasa, the cosmic ether, and Prana energy. When Prana acts upon Akasa all forms of matter are created. This idea corresponds broadly to that of modern nuclear physics, which regards all matter as energy 'organised' in different ways. Magnetism is a manifestation of Prana, so are electricity and gravitation. Everything in the universe that moves is a manifestation of Prana. Thanks to Prana the wind blows, the earth trembles, an aeroplane takes off, a star explodes. We exist in an ocean of Prana where everything is vortex. Yogis affirm that what characterises life is its ability to attack Prana to itself, to store it up and transform it for influence upon both the inner and outer world.

According to the yogis, Prana is present in the atmosphere, yet it is neither oxygen, nor nitrogen, nor any other chemical constituent of the atmosphere. Prana exists in our food, water, sunlight, but it is neither vitamin nor warmth nor ultraviolet rays. Air, water, and food, sunlight: all convey the Prana on which all animals and vegetable life depends. Prana penetrates the whole body, even where the air cannot reach. Prana is our true nourishment, for without Prana, there can be no life." Prana to a yogi is electricity of the modern civilisation.

Let us suppose for a moment that we have been taken back two thousand years ago and we are trying to explain to a yogi what our own way of life is like, with its, telephone, radio, television, refrigerators, motor cars, aeroplanes, vacuum cleaner, satellites and space rockets, electronic lamps etc. etc., without mentioning their driving force, electricity. He would understand nothing of its basic driving force, which we use without thinking much about it. It is possible and useful to practice asana without knowing the essence of Prana. The yogic postures automatically use Prana in the body. Once the techniques of asana are mastered, then, material and mechanical exercises of asana reach the stage of applying the Prana doing Pranayama. Pranayama is the most vital of sciences since ultimately all energies which show them in the form of life are pranic, Every human being from life to death handles prana without, however, being involved in pranayama. The first objective of Pranayama is to store the bioelectrical energy and direct and distribute it at will in the body to gain control by our mental consciousness for our physical and mental health. We exist by constantly drawing Prana from cosmos using the nerve ending in the nasal cavities, the air cells in the lungs, the tongue and our skin. The yogis regard the nose as the main Prana absorbing organ. Our nose cavities has infinite numbers of ultra-sensitive nervous receptors which automatically the qualitative variations of the air. We can differentiate a bad smell and soothing good scent of flower or perfume. In case of bad smell, the body immediately becomes alert. The senility of our nasal receptors is incredible. A pleasant smell encourages us to breathe deeply.

According to Dr. J Valnet, Hospital, Paris, 1961, says: In aromatherapy the natural plant essence... "Carried by the blood stream, the ionised plant aroma impregnates every corner of the body, powerfully vitalises the polarised and discharge cells, replenishes electronic shortages by recharging the bioelectrical batteries, and disperses the cellular residue by dissolving the viscous and diseased substances of body fluids. It oxidises the poisonous metabolic waste products, increases the energy balance, frees the mechanism of organic oxidation, and of self-regulation, and reaches the lungs and kidneys whence it is exhaled or extracts without trace. The powerful electrolytic charges of the aroma, by cleansing the cells, restart the wave of vibration and re-establish the electro-sanguine exchanges within and between the tissues". Most of us already know the use of smelling salt when someone faints. In fact, when someone is fainted and barely breathing. the use of smelling salt helps the victim to breathe again. The nostrils are in reflex contact with whole nervous mechanism of the body to control our bodily functions.

Similarly, the nostrils are the main organs of Prana (air cells or alveoli) absorption and transfer the Pranic energy (Oxygen) to the lungs, the passage of Oxygen from alveoli into the blood. According to yogis, the tongue is also an important organ which absorbs Prana energy from food which identifies taste. Our skin is also the largest and most important organ of the body which can absorb a large quantity of radiant solar Prana energy. According to yogis the absorption and accumulation of Prana energy are also controlled by our thoughts.

CHAPTER THREE

Preliminaries of Pranayama Yoga

3.1 Consideration of age

The wide general observation by ancient authorities affirm that not only the young and old but even the very old and sick can undertake the practice of Pranayama yoga with success to achieve the highest benefit thereof. However, to practice the physical yoga and Pranayama need to be regulated with great care in relation to the age of an individual. In childhood the diameter of arteries and the volume of the heart is proportionately smaller than it is later on. The volume of the heart is generally increased twelvefold during adolescence; the heart is still quite unprepared to withstand the strain, hence unusual physical exertion should be regulated.

Children under the age of five years should not be initiated in to Pranayama yoga exercises, their natural movements and play being considered sufficient for the harmonic growth of various organs and parts of the body. It is advised from the beginning of the tenth to the end of the sixteenth year when it is really the time for most rapid growth both in height and weight and their cortical area of the brain are fast developing should be encouraged to daily systematic exercise. There is also substantiated scientific evidence that moderate and regular exercise stimulates a normalising of important endocrine secretion which contributes to health and well-being.

From this point of view, much additional benefit from Pranayama yoga exercise may be gained by the conscious association of the mind to the varying movements of the body. When practiced with absolute regularity, the mental effort will synchronise automatically with each muscle that moves in every exercise and the exercises themselves will soon grow into the daily habits of life for maximum benefit.

What needs to be impressed however is that when, as too often happens, the daily dose of exercise is missed. In such cases the exercise should be made good as soon as possible at some other time of the day or, at the least, the next day. This is extremely essential to maintain the daily health rhythm and consequently the wholesome equilibrium of well-rounded hygienic life. In short, as far as possible, whenever the opportunity for yoga exercise is missed for one reason or another, the balance must be restored quickly by an extra dose the very next day for the maximum benefit.

CHAPTER FOUR

Science of Pranayama

The existence of Prana and to be able to control has been justified by many yogis and scientists. For instance experiments have been carried out on the spot by Dr.Therese Brosse, with simultaneous pneumographic and cardio graphic recordings. The extract of her published reports says:

"Just when the yogi announces that his heart is under control only the minutes fibrillation is visible on the iso-electric graph, the merest trace of cardiac contraction and almost impossible to record. On seeing this trace it would be possible to reach the most serious prognosis were it not that, in the moments immediately before and after, the recorded line is not only normal but even exaggerated in voltage at the will of the yogi......" "faced with such facts it is of little importance that we attribute them to an abnormal concentration of carbon dioxide in the blood, to a change of the heart's axis, to a modification of tissue ionisation, to a combination of all these processes or others unsuspected of which the present state of our knowledge does not permit us to take account. Whatever it might be, it remains truly astonishing that the extreme fall in voltage takes place precisely when the yogi announces that he is about to withdraw the vital energy from his heart, and that the voltage returns to normal or above it when he claims that he is in control of the normal functioning of his heart. To the mind of yogi the vital energy (Prana) is an electrical energy which he declares is of the same nature as lighting. On the other hand it is by a special science of breathing that he means to regulate that vital energy, at least that which he draws from nature. Quite recent works have made clear the role of the lungs so far as electrical change in the blood is concerned, the alveoli extracting the negative ions from the inhaled air, which pass on their vitality to the colloids"

"Thus we find ourselves in the presence of men with an almost complete mastery of the various human activities and who, without any knowledge of structure of their organs, can master their functions nonetheless. Moreover, they enjoy magnificent health which they could not maintain if they were ceaselessly violating physiological laws during their extraordinary and prolonged exercises. As we have just seen, the very theory on which some of these exercises are based seems to be confirmed, not only by the results but also by recent discoveries by scientific tests".

According to Dr. Therese Brosse "yogi when controls his heart and even stops it, is of the same nature of lightning and affirms that the Prana in the atmosphere is composed if, not completely at least fundamentally, of electrically charged particles, negative ions in fact, and also that a true metabolism takes place within our bodies of the electricity we draw from the atmosphere and the ionisation of the air consists of short-wave electromagnetic radiation from that inexhaustible generator of electricity, the sun. Cosmic rays are another source. While the sun's rays are restricted during night or, rays blocked by cloud, the cosmic rays are continuously active and penetrate the thickest layers of cloud without losing any of their energy. One of the aims of Pranayama, amongst others, is to enable to fix more of this energy, to store, to distribute within the organism, and to direct it wherever the need is felt."

Regulation of breath control has many different purposes. Any time is a good time to control one's breathing. No matter, how many times we practice breathe awareness, one stressful situation can cause us to lose control of our breathing. When we have no control over our breathing, our blood pressure may also follow suit. When our breath is out of control, the mind will also be out of balance.

It is therefore, important to understand the effect of yoga and pranayama on the human body and also how the internal systems of the body including anatomical and physiological descriptions of various organs of the body operate. As far as practicable, the medical terminologies have been omitted as these may be properly studied through authoritative texts.

4.1: Internal systems of the body

There are basically six main systems of the body together with mental hygiene. The main systems of the body those are important and useful for practicing yoga and Pranayama have been described. Those are:

4.1.1) The Circulatory system
4.1.2) The Respiratory system
4.1.3) The Endocrine system
4.1.4) The Digestive system
4.1.5) The Nervous system and
4.1.6) Mental hygiene
4.1.7) How to practice
4.1.1) The Circulatory system

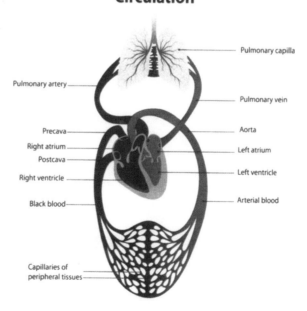

Figure 1

In our body, the heart, blood, arteries, veins and capillaries are the component parts of the circulatory system. Each part has its own function. For example, arteries are simple tubes that carry blood away from the heart. Veins are also tubes that help to return blood to the heart. The blood performs very important part, without it we cannot survive. Blood is pumped by the heart through the network of tubes to all parts of the body. The heart is like a pump which continuously working, as long we are alive. Capillaries are tiny tubes that connect the arteries and veins. Their main function is to exchange and clear out waste between blood cells The circulatory system works in three ways- the pulmonary circulation, which the movement of blood between the lungs and the heart; Coronary circulation, which is the movement of blood within the heart chambers and systematic circulation, which moves the blood from the heart to the rest of the body. For our body to function properly the blood has to reach in every parts of the body. Yoga and Pranayama plays a great part to do just that.

4.1.2: The Respiratory system

The respiratory centre of the brain controls the respiratory system. This system also controls and regulates the respiratory muscles so that the right amount of air goes in our lung to suit our activities. There are two types of neurons (nerve cells) alternately control our rate of breathing in and out functions. Although it is a voluntary movement, yet we cannot stop ourselves breathing all together. The respiratory centre of the brain (cerebral cortex) over rides the brain and takes control of our breathing.

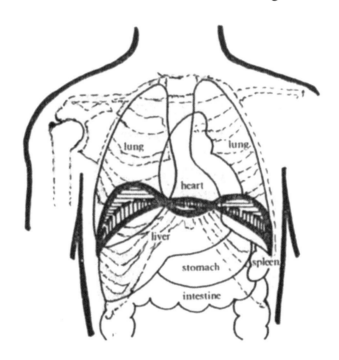

Figure 2

Breathing is normally done by our nose, although, it is easier to breathe through our mouth. However, it is healthy to breathe through our nose. Inside the nose, the nasal hair and mucus act as a filter. This filter protects dirt or impurities to get inside the lung. The thin bone in side our nose warms the air by friction as it comes in. The air we breathe in goes from our nose through the windpipe to the lung. The flap at the upper end of the trachea, protect the food getting into the lung. There are two short branches at the end of the trachea, called bronchi. They branch out into very small tubes are called bronchioles. At the end of the bronchioles there are clusters of sacs called alveoli. When we breathe, oxygen and carbon dioxide gets separated between the alveoli and its surrounding capillaries. Our diaphragm helps to move the air in and out of the lung. The diaphragm and the abdominal muscles control the amount of air pressure required in the chest when we breathe in. The nerves around the lung, sends information to the brain that regulates the rhythm of breathing and also detects the amount of carbon dioxide in the blood. Depending on the amount of carbon dioxide present in the blood the brain signals the diaphragm to increase or decrease its size for intake of oxygen and the breathing rate. Yoga breathing exercises voluntarily control the intake of air there by controlling the oxygen intake in the lung.

4.1.3: The Endocrine system

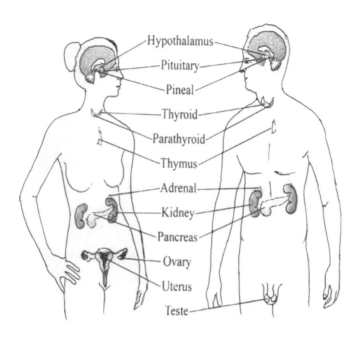

Figure 3

These are system of glands in the body. These glands release the chemical hormones transported directly to the blood stream, to different organs and tissues and cells of the body. Each kind of hormone affects only to its target cells. These glands produce more than 20 types of chemical hormones. The variation of hormone levels varies in the body and influences stress level, infection, and the balance of fluid and minerals in the blood. The functions of the endocrine system are very important for our body. A variety of disorders can arise if the endocrine system doesn't function properly. Yoga exercises and Pranayama are designed to specifically activate certain glands for their proper functions. In this section, only the simple functions of glands are mentioned without going too much into medical details.

The main glands are: Hypothalamus, Pineal gland, Pituitary gland, Thyroid gland, Para-thyroid gland, Adrenal gland, Pancreas gland and Ovary or the reproductive gland for women. The controlling of all the glands is carried out by the Hypothalamus located in the lower central part of the brain. It controls the Pituitary gland, which is located in the base of the brain. The secretion of hormones of the pituitary gland controls other glands and other parts of the body. Such as growth hormones produced by the pituitary gland through lever promotes growth of the body. In female body, through mammary gland, controls the milk production of the body after the childbirth. Through ovary, controls the reproductive functions of the body and through kidney, controls the water retention of the body. The pituitary gland also secretes hormones that act on the nervous system to reduce sensitivity to pain, and signal the ovaries to make sex hormones, and that control ovulation and the menstrual cycle as well as the contractions in the uterus that occur during labour in women.

The next important gland is the Thyroid gland. This gland is located in the neck at the lower part of the larynx. The hormone produced by this gland regulates the growth of the body. Over activity of this gland can cause increase in respiration, rise in body temperature consequently increase in blood pressure. On the other hand under activity of this produces the opposite effects.

Parathyroid glands are located one on top of each kidney. It has two parts and each part produces hormones; one regulates salt and water balance in the body together with the body's response to stress, the immune system, and the sexual function of the body. The other part produces hormones that increase heart rate and blood pressure when we are under stress.

The pineal gland is located in the middle of the brain. It secretes a hormone that regulates our wake and sleep cycle. The pancreas gland produces hormones, which maintains and balances sugar level in the blood there by controls the energy level in the body.

4.1.4: The Digestive system

The digestion is a process by which food is broken down into smaller and smaller parts. They eventually carry them through to blood system for nourishment of various parts of the body. The digestive system basically consists of a long tube connected from our mouth to the anus. Along the way the tube is connected to various organs of the body such as mouth, stomach, small and large intestines and colon. The mechanical and chemical digestive process begins in the mouth when the food is chewed. When we swallow the food the chewed food goes into our stomach. From here the involuntary chemical process of further digestion continues under the control of various nerves. Our stomach naturally produces gastric juice and by automatic muscular action churns the food and further breaks them down into separate chemicals as it travel down the tube.

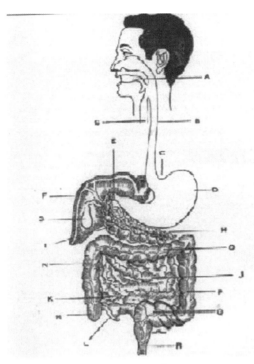

Figure 4

A- Mouth, B-Esophagua, C-Abdominal part, D- Stomach, E-Opening of Stomach
F-Liver, G-Gallbladder, H-Pancreas, I- Pancriatic duct, J-Small Intestine
K- Eleuns L-Appendix, M-Cecum, N- Ascending Colon, O- Transverse Colon
P-Large Intestine, Q-Sigmoid Colon, R-Anus Canal, S -Breathing Canal

The waste products that are undigested parts of the food such as fibres are pushed down into the colon and eventually the faeces are expelled from our body by bowl movement. However, the digested molecules of food as well as water, minerals and vitamins from the diet are absorbed from the cavity of the upper small intestine and eventually go into our blood stream for the nourishment of the body.

The system seems to be very simple; however, our body has to produce the correct chemicals of the correct amount to breakdown protein, fat, and carbohydrate of our food that we consume. The malfunction of any of these glands can cause digestive problems or digestive related diseases.

Yoga and Pranayama exercises are especially designed to improve the basic process of digestion and the function of the major digestive organs. General consensus of some health professional indicates that if not all, a number of major diseases start in the colon due to malfunction or imbalance of our endocrine system. Some experts assert that basically there are two main reasons of diseases in human body.

Poor function of the circulatory system that causes unwanted toxins to accumulate in the body. Imbalance and uncoordinated activities of muscular, endocrine, digestive and psychological are the basic cause of diseases. Most of our food that we consume has some form of preservatives, artificial ingredients, genetically engineered chemicals and activities. They all contribute to our present ever-increasing gastrointestinal health crisis and most of them are related to colon function of the body. It is therefore very important to improve our digestive and assimilation process and clear out old accumulation of waste from our intestinal track. The overall digestive process is also related to our immune system of the body. The proper function of the endocrine system will certainly improve our immune system. The lack of coordination between these processes is the root cause of all diseases. Yoga and pranayama exercises therefore, are most effective and preventive tool to attain a perfect balance of the internal system of our body. A far as the digestive system is concerned, the types of food we consume are also very important.

Therefore, control of the abdomen is also very important for pranayama. It helps to increase the active behaviour of the abdominal wall which in turn affects the respiratory process of the body. The active behaviour and control of abdominal muscles at will helps to improve the respiratory system of the lung and the function of the liver.

4.1.5: The Nervous system

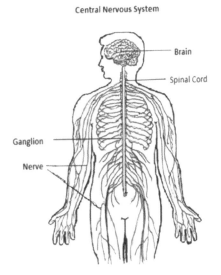

Central Nervous System

Brain

Spinal Cord

Ganglion

Nerve

Figure 5

The nervous system is the most complex system of our body. This system gathers stores and interprets information and controls them. This system uses electrical impulses that travel along the length of one nerve cell (neurons) to another. These neurons process the information within a milli-second initiate action through sensory or motor nerves. This system controls and coordinates all essential of the human body. Basically the nervous system has four main functions:

1. To gather information from outside or inside the body.
2. To transmit information back and forth through the brain and the spinal cord.
3. To process information for the best response.
4. To send information to muscles, glands and different organs of the body for their correct response.

It acts voluntarily as well as involuntarily. The system has two major divisions:

The central nervous system consists of brain and the spinal cord where the spinal cord provides the link between the brain and the rest of the body. It is like a control centre of information.

The Peripheral nervous system though connected to the central nervous system is located outside the spinal cord and the brain. It had two divisions the sensory and the motor divisions. The voluntary nervous system relays information from skin and muscles whereas the automatic involuntary nervous system relays information to internal organs. The involuntary system also works in two ways.

1. The sympathetic nervous system that controls our organs in time of stress and fear.
2. The Parasympathetic nervous system, that controls when our body is at rest.

There are three main components of the brain, namely the brainstem, cerebellum and the forebrain. For the purpose of yoga, in this section only the simple function of fore brain has been explained. The activities of the Fore brain are divided into many component parts. Each one is very important to understand as far as the yoga exercises are concerned. The component parts of forebrain are:

1. The Hypothalamus
2. The Cerebrum and Cerebral cortex.

The cerebral cortex is also divided into four parts namely Frontal lobe, Parietal lobe, Temporal lobe and the Occipital lobe. The frontal lobe is located near the temple and forehead. It controls our speech, tongue and voluntary muscle movements. The proper function of this lobe is important to be able to do yoga postures.

The Parietal lobe is situated behind the frontal lobe and it deals with awareness. Self-awareness is a very important part of yoga meditative exercises.

The Temporal lobe is located parallel to our ears and it deals with sound reception and the Occipital lobe controls our eye functions. The proper functions of all these lobes are very important to be able to do the yoga exercises.

The brain performs an incredible number of tasks. It is beyond the scope of this book to mention the complicated function of the brain. However, it must be emphasized that yoga exercises help to attain the proper function of all the parts of the brain. Our body balance for instance, is done by the cerebellum, which controls the contractions of muscles necessary to maintain a balance. Yoga practice helps not only to get the physical balance but also helps to improve the immune system of the body. Yoga postures together with pranayama (breathing) and relaxation techniques relax the nervous system. It is a powerful tool to help stimulate or calm the immune response of the body. Since health of every tissue in the body depends upon the health of brain and spine, yoga plays a greater role in gaining vitality of the spine and rejuvenation of mind. Most yoga exercises are especially designed to improve the function of the spine and the activity of the brain.

4.1.6: Mental hygiene

Our body and mind are very much related. It is said that a healthy body has a healthy mind. However, like the way we need to train our body to be healthy, we need to train our mind as well. In this section simple yoga techniques are mentioned to improve the mental faculty. Examples are given that will help to gain will power using visualization techniques, to analyse and to understand our inner mind, overcome fear and also develop mental power, imagination and positive attitude to encourage positive living life style. The destructive emotions cause jealously, possessiveness, demanding attitude and insecurity. Mental exercises together with yoga exercises will help to overcome such negative emotions. For that it is necessary to learn and train our mind. Mental exercises are not so easy. It takes a lot of practice to master them. Some people find it easy to discipline their minds easily whereas others may struggle a lot to concentrate to control their minds.

According to yoga there are five types of mind such as: The conscious mind that we can control if we want consciously. The sub-conscious mind, that works on its own based on our experiences in life that can only be reached by training. The para-conscious mind is the transition between the conscious and the subconscious minds, when we dream to release our mental tension. The sub-conscious mind when both our conscious and the unconscious mind are inactive. The super-conscious mind, that we do not know much about which beyond the scope of this book. Mental exercises can be done anywhere and at any time but to achieve quick results we should always practice at a time and place, which is least distractive.

4.1.7: How to practice

Irrespective of individual's interest whether in physical training, mental discipline or spiritual realisation, preference in the Pranayama yoga exercises are given first and always to the proficiency in any one meditative posture for composure, ease, breathing and concentration. In all, there are twenty-eight meditative postures of sitting. Notwithstanding the old tradition which regarded Siddhasana or the (Perfect-pose) and Padmasana or the (Lotus –pose) as classic poses suited to meditation. However, the easy-pose (Sukhasana) or the Lotus pose (Padmasan) as the classical poses for Pranayama

i: Sukhasana (The Easy pose or Cross-legged posture:

Sit in a comfortable cross-legged posture (Sukhasana) as shown in figure 6, close your eyes, make your body completely relaxed and breathe slowly and rhythmically. This will help you to get complete stillness of mind particularly when thoughts are wondering about from one thought to other in your mind.

Do not get distracted if you find difficult to avoid thoughts rushing about in your mind. Try to concentrate and visualise anything or any object in your mind such as: flower, cloud, your son, daughter, or husband or wife's picture. Try to hold on to the picture several minutes. At first you may find it very difficult to hold on to the picture in your mind for too long but with practice you will find that it isn't so difficult.

There are several recommended sitting postures. All have specific benefits for specific parts of the body. Each sitting posture and its benefits is explained in brief. You may find it difficult to do some of the exercises such as the Lotus posture, particularly if you have short legs and heavy thighs. Do not despair and feel dejected. Other sitting postures will give you equally added benefits.

All sitting postures are designed to get a perfect balance of the body while sitting. These postures help to breathe easily thereby getting more oxygen in the lungs to purify the blood. They naturally help to keep the back straight. Depending on the requirements, the sitting postures generally restrict the flow of blood in the legs by putting pressure on pressure points of the legs thereby slowing down the blood flow in the leg. After sitting in a sitting posture you should straighten your legs for blood to flow freely in all parts of your legs. This will have a flushing effect on arteries of the legs.

All sitting postures with slow and deep breathing help to develop concentration, inner strength and courage. Posture such as the Lotus posture also opens up the knee joints that help to avoid arthritis, a common illness at an older age.

In modern houses, we tend to sit comfortably either on a chair or a settee, however, this does not give the legs the exercises needed. Our legs get tired standing for the whole day and taking all the weight of our body, therefore the legs need proper nourishment.

The Easy pose,(Sukhasana) as shown in figure 6, as the name suggests, is the easiest of all postures. Simply sit with legs crossed, keeping your back and neck in a straight line and resting your hands on your knees.

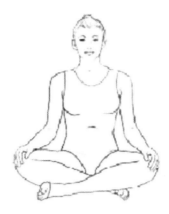

Figure 6. Sukhasana (the Easy Pose or Crossed leg posture)

ii: Siddhasana (the Pose of an Adept or Perfect posture:

This posture is sometimes known as the perfect posture. It helps to tone up all the nerve centres around the pelvic region. This posture balances the body perfectly. Pelvic bones take up the body weight when the spine is kept erect. At this posture, all the internal organs rest at the correct position. This posture aids in breathing effectively thereby helps to purify the blood. The restriction of the flow of blood around the legs helps more blood to reach the upper parts of the body especially to all the nerve centres and the head. This is a good position for developing concentration as well. (See figure 7)

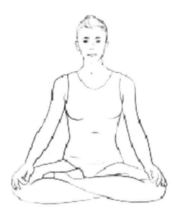

Figure 7. Siddhasana, (Pose of an Adept)

How to practice

i). Sit on the ground spreading both legs straight on front of you keeping them together then bend the right leg and bring the heel of the leg close to the thigh of the left leg.

ii). Bend the left leg and place the foot in the crease formed by the right thigh and the calf of the right leg so that the calf of the left leg is on top of the right toe.

iii). Place both hands on the top of your knees.

iv). Stay in this position for a while and repeat the same posture using opposite legs so that the left leg is at the bottom and the right leg is on the top.

iii:. Ardha Padmasana (The Half Lotus Posture:

Half lotus posture has the similar benefits of a Full lotus posture but to a lesser extent. A Full lotus postures is difficult to do, particularly, those who have short legs and heavy thighs. Some of you may find it almost impossible to perform the Full lotus position because of the way your legs and the hip joints are set. In that case, you find it difficult to do the Full lotus posture, they should try to do the half lotus position. (See figure 8a & 8b).

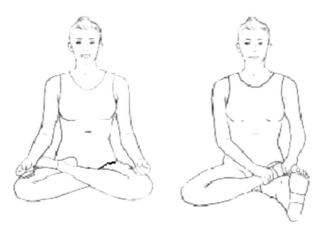

Figure 8b   Figure 8a
(The Half Lotus posture)

How to practice

i).   Sit on the ground spreading both legs straight on front of you keeping them together. Bend the right leg and bring the right heel close to the left groin in order to apply pressure on the arteries near the groin.

ii).   Bend the left leg and place the left foot over the right thigh.

iii). Stay in this position for a while and repeat the same posture using opposite legs so that the right foot is placed over the left thigh.

iv:. Padmasana (The Lotus Posture:

For this posture both legs are inter locked with both the heels touching the groin. Both heels put pressure on the main arteries near the groin. The effect of this increased pressure restricts the flow of blood circulation in the legs and directs the blood supply to the upper parts of the body and the head. This posture is considered to be the best posture for meditation and concentration. The Lotus posture can also help to develop confidence, tranquillity and poise. This posture relaxes your body and mind quickly.(See figure 9a & 9b)

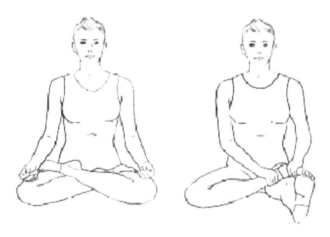

Figure 9a   **Figure 9b**
(The Lotus Posture)

How to practice

i).   Sit on the ground spreading both legs straight on front of you keeping them together. Bend the left leg and bring the left heel close to the right groin placing the foot onto the right thigh.

ii).   Bend the right leg and grab your right toe with your hand and place the right foot over the left thigh so that the knees are touching the ground.

iii). Stay in this position for a while and repeat the same posture using opposite legs so that the right foot is placed onto the left thigh and vice versa.

iv).   When completed lift your leg using your hands and straighten one leg at a time to resume the starting position.

v:. Muktasana (The Free Pose:

In this posture both legs are folded and brought one in front of the other. However, both knees are placed flat on the ground. This may be difficult in some cases to place your knees flat on the ground but with some practice, when your joints become flexible, you will be able to do this exercise easily. This posture helps to slacken and lubricate the pelvic joints and also helps to spread the knees wide apart. (see figure 10)

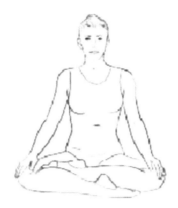

Figure 10 Muktasana (The free pose)

How to practice

i). Sit on the ground spreading both legs straight on front of you keeping them together.
ii). Bend both legs towards the body so that both are lying next to each other side by side.
iii). Place your palms on both knees and put pressure on your knees flat on the ground.
iv). Stay in this position for a while then straighten your legs and relax.

CHAPTER FIVE

Breathing Techniques of Pranayama

Breathing is a natural thing for all human being. No one can live for more than few minutes without breathing. Most people use only a fraction of their full breathing capacity. We breathe 28 differently at different times depending on our requirements of the body. For instance if we run, we breathe faster because more purified blood is needed at different parts of the body and our heart starts to pump faster. To purify the blood we need more oxygen therefore we breathe faster. The opposite of that is, when we are relaxed and lie down in bed, or asleep we tend to breathe slowly.

Proper breathing helps to eliminate tensions and develops positive mental attitudes. Most of us develop bad breathing habits due to a combination of many factors such as stress, poor posture and wrong sitting habits. All yoga- breathing exercises have the effect of increasing the amount of air, which enters the lungs and purifies the blood. In pranayama yoga breathing, proper exhalation is absolutely a prerequisite of correct and complete inhalation. Unless we breathe out fully it is impossible to breathe in properly.

Pranayama yogic breathing, works in three phases in which all parts of the lungs is filled with air into one simple and full rhythmic movement in a continuous flow without gasping. The three phases of yoga breathing are:

1. Diaphragmatic or abdominal breathing
2. Intercostal breathing where rib cage is expanded
3. Breathing from the top of the lungs produced by raising the collar without raising the shoulders and the upper part of the thorax.

In pranayama yoga breathing all three sequences should be done in conjunction. Breathing should be deep, slow, silent, continuous and easy. Always breathe through your nose unless instructed except in a particular type of breathing where the mouth or teeth breathing are used. Concentrate your mind entirely upon the action of breathing. Do not blow yourself like a balloon. In pranayama yoga breathing, inhalation exhalation should be carried out in slow and complete relaxed state. There should be no strain in any muscles. You should not hear yourself breathe. During exhalation the stomach muscles should be contracted so as to help the lungs to empty the air to their full extent. Although there is always a residue of impure air that remains in the lung during exhalation, you must attempt to minimize the residue of impure air so that you can breathe in more fresh air during inhalation.

Proper breathing will provide sufficient oxygen to purify the blood for the correct and efficient functioning of the body cells. While exhaling we breathe out carbon dioxide. We need proper supply of oxygen in our lungs. Lack of oxygen in our breathing will result in fatigue, confusion, sluggishness, and loss of mental balance, concentration, memory and the control of emotions. Proper yoga breathing will help you to keep the two sides of your brain in balance. However during breathing exercise, do not hold your breath for too long unless you are guided by an experienced yoga teacher. Do not practice cleansing or dynamic version of breathing if you are suffering from heart condition or hernia.

It is very important to understand the aerodynamic peculiarity of our nose to practice Pranayama. The respiratory centre of the brain controls the respiratory system. This system also controls and regulates the respiratory muscles so that the right amount of air goes in our lung to suit our activities. There are two types of neurons (nerve cells) alternately control our rate of breathing in and out functions. Although it is a voluntary movement, yet, we cannot stop ourselves breathing all together. The respiratory centre of the brain (cerebral cortex) over rides the brain and takes control of our breathing. This in turn gets the greatest possible quantity of Prana in the brain. Normally, we all know that we breathe differently at different times such as: when running, sleeping or relaxing. There are correlations between our breathing in our physical, intellectual and emotional activities. In Pranayama breathing techniques, the length of breathing, duration of breathing and rhythm of breathing are controlled according to our particular needs. The yogic name of the left nostril is called 'Ida'(cooling nostril) while the right nostril is called 'Pingala'(warming nostril). The nostrils are the main organs of Prana absorption and the lungs are the seat of important Pranic activities of the air cells (alveoli) of the lungs. The bioelectric system of the lung uses the oxygen from the alveoli into the blood. When we have concentrated thoughts, we absolve larger amount of Prana. Our mind can therefore direct the absorption, storage, control and distribution of Prana in our body. The Pranayama, such as Nadi Shodhana, where alter net breathing exercise is carried out for purifying the Nadi, (subtle channels through which energy of Prana flows). For this breathing technique, our both nostrils play unique roles and they should be free and clear. We know that our one or other nostril is often blocked (alternate rhinitis) and this is quite normal and this alternation of blocked nose occurs continuously during the day with lesser or greater intensity which generally unnoticed. (See Figure 11, the Chakras).

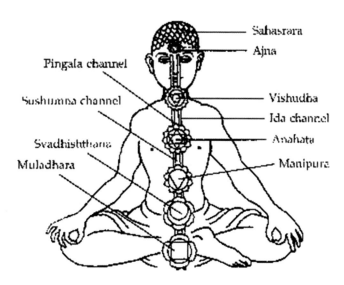

Figure 11. The Chakras

Pranayama is a method to balance and equalise the Pranic current flowing through the nose to purify the whole network of Nadis (tubes in Sanskrit) through which our energy flows. The yogis found by their internal perception, have noticed that the circulation of energy within their bodies along Nadis. This subtle physiology is based on their internal observation and portrayed the Nadis graphically and the positions of these vital points so called Chakras as shown in the Figure 11

The Pranayama exercise tries to harness these two sets of currents, and by making them unite to still both body and mind. Pranayama breathing exercises are all designed to create the uniting of these two currents. The concentration of energy is pushed down to the base of the spine. Here there is situated one of the seven chakras of the body and the entrance of the Susumna, the spinal canal.

The positions of this representation, the yogis, know and say that Chakras are situated in the body. Chakras though cannot be taken as a strict anatomical presentation. The experienced yogis assert that these Chakras exist in our body like a coiled-up snake in a state of hibernation, and remains asleep near the lower extremity of person's backbone is called Kundalini in Sanskrit, means something is coiled up such as a snake. According to the experienced yogis there are thousands of Nadis which serve as carriers of Prana. Among all the Nadis, ten are particularly noteworthy. The human backbone or spinal column there are two parallel Nadis passing through channels, the left channel is called 'Ida' and the right channel is called 'Pingala' According to experience yogis when we exhale the breath is stronger through the left nostril, and it indicates that our vital energy is flowing through the 'Ida' channel . Similarly, if the breath is stronger through his right nostril, then the energy is flowing through the 'Pingala channel. It is also said that when a person does heavy physical activity, his energy flows through the 'Pingala' channel and when resting the energy flows through the 'Ida' channel. According the yogis there is a third channel inside the backbone between the 'Ida' and 'Pingala' is called 'Susumna'. Normally the 'Susumna' channel remains dormant and it opens up when the kundalini power is awakened i.e. channels towards the brain passing through several different doors and each of these doors or level of spiritual experience is called a 'Chakrsa'. According to Raja yoga philosophy, seven such levels exist in the path of spinal column. The top most one is named 'Sahasrara' which is located somewhere inside the brain. The lowest one, which is situated at the lower end of spinal cord, is called 'Muladhara'. The next higher Chakra is 'Svadhisthana', and then comes 'Manipura', 'Anahata', 'Vishuddha', 'Ajna', and 'Sahasrara'. According to experienced Yogis when Kundalini power reaches the Sahasrara through the Susumna channel, the yogi reaches the goal of Yoga. For all practical purposes, unless we are expecting to get the ultimate reward of Pranayama through Raja Yoga practice, we can get all the benefits of guaranteed excellent health. "For most people, the Susumna is never opened, as long as they live. However, according to experienced yogi, by directing energy through the Susumna, the yogi finds that the spiritual life has become all at once much easier and a whole range of spiritual options opens themselves to him"

The ultimate goal of Pranayama is to gain Samadhi. In the words of Swami Vivekananda, a past master of Raja Yoga, "to get to that stage of Samadhi, there must be perfect chastity, in thought, word, and deed."

Generally, you may notice while practicing pranayama, the air current is not identical on both nostrils. If one nostril is severely blocked and preventing to breathe effectively with that nostril, then, it is necessary to clear the nostril. For instant, suppose your left nostril is blocked, then, to clear the nostril you should lie down on your right side and relax for a few minutes, you will notice that the blocked nostril is clearing and the air is passing freely, while the right nostril remains clear because the prime objectives of Pranayama is to ensure a free circulation of pranic forces at all levels.

The second technique to clear the blocked nostril is to find a spot at the back of neck near the base of the skull and a gentle but firm pressure on this spot will clear the blocked nostril. Generally, despite this cleansing, one or other nostril often noticed partly blocked. This is quite normal, the obstruction passes from one nostril to other approximately every two hours, called in medical term as "alternate rhinitis" which usually goes unnoticed.

After clearing the blocked nostril, the alternate breathing may be practice in any of the sitting postures mentioned earlier.

5.1: Simple Breathing Exercises & their Benefits

There are several simple breathing exercises those can be practiced which calms and balances the mind and body, aids relaxation, improves concentration, strengthens and increases the respiration capacity. It also helps to overcome insomnia, stress and anxiety. These exercises can be practiced at anytime and anywhere. This exercise helps to relax your body and mind quickly.

For example:

5.1.1: Breathing to eliminate anxiety.

This exercise is very useful for eliminating mental anxiety very quickly. It acts as an antidote to help panic attack. You can practice this exercise at anytime and anywhere. This exercise can be done while sitting, standing or lying down.

How to practice

i).   Sit comfortable in a crossed-legged position. Relax your facial muscles and breathe
ii). Inhale deeply and slowly through both nostrils without any strain.
iii). Exhale very slowly and steadily concentrating above your navel area.
iv). Inhale again and increase the inhalation and exhalation time gradually.
v).   Repeat the exercise a few times.
vi). On completion, resume normal breathing and relax.

5.1.2: Breathing to eliminate pain. (Visualization breathing:

This exercise works on the principle of breathing with visualizing the area of pain. When you visualize your affected area with pain an extra supply of oxygen with prana is directed to that specific area. The technique is to inhale and visualize the prana accumulating in the solar plexus (area just above the navel).

How to practice

i).   Sit comfortably in a crossed-legged position and breathe normally.
ii). Hold your breath for a while then exhale and concentrate on the area of pain as if prana is directed towards the affected area-
iii). If you can touch the area of pain by your fingers then think, as if the pain-relieving energy is flowing through your arms to the fingertip and taking the pain away.
iv). Repeat the exercise a few times. Breathe normally and relax.

5.1.3: Simple Breathing to calm & ventilate the lungs:

The simple cleansing breath calms and ventilates the lungs. It helps to tone up the body, releases stress and frustrations quickly. This exercise can be done while sitting or standing.

How to practice

i). Sit comfortably in a crossed-legged position. Close your eyes, relax your face muscles and breathe normally.

ii). Inhale through both nostrils slowly, smoothly and deeply without any strain on your facial and neck muscles.

iii). Hold your breath for a little while; shape your lips as if you are going to whistle.

iv). Exhale through your mouth forcefully with a steady stream of air blowing out of your mouth. Do not puff.

v). Expel the air until the lung is completely empty.

vi). Repeat the exercise a few times.

vii). Resume normal breathing.

5.1.4: Dynamic Breathing for cleansing the respiratory passage. .

This is an excellent exercise for cleansing the respiratory passage. It strengthens the abdominal muscles, abdominal organs and stimulates lung tissues. It helps to improve the nervous system of the body.

How to practice

i). Sit comfortably in a crossed-legged position. Close your eyes and relax your body and arms.

ii). Inhale with both nostrils slowly, deeply and without any strain.

iii). Exhale in a short burst, and at the same time tighten your stomach muscles.

iv). Inhale again which will follow naturally.

v). Repeat this exercise a few times

vi). Resume normal breathing and relax.

5.1.5: Three part Breathing to purify blood.

This exercise teaches you to fill up the chambers of your lungs effectively. It begins with the stomach breathing, moving up through the lower ribcage to the upper part of the lungs. This exercise promotes proper breathing sequence for yoga exercise. It relaxes the mind and body. It purifies the blood and helps to eliminate carbon dioxide from the lung. This exercise can be done sitting down or lying down during yoga exercise or any time you feel like.

How to Practice

    i).   Sit comfortably in a crossed-legged position or lie down on your back with your legs slightly vapart. Relax your body and arms by your sides

    ii).   Begin taking long, slow, deep breaths through both nostrils.

    iii).   Inhale and allow your stomach to fill with air. Slowly draw- air into the lower part of the lungs and then inflate the upper part by moving your collar bones.

    iv).   Exhale by allowing your stomach to deflate a balloon.

    v).   Repeat this exercise slowly, several times using the same sequence.

    vi).   On completion relax, your arms and hands and breathe normally.

5.1.6: Sigh Breathing to remove congestion of the chest.

This is a very useful exercise when you have congestion in your chest and you find it difficult to breathe. It also assists to relieve tension and stress. Breathe in short bursts and breathe out using a steady flow.

How to Practice

    i).   Sit comfortable in a crossed-legged position, close your eyes and relax.

    ii).   Inhales using short quick bursts but not a continuous inhalation through your mouth.

    iii).   Exhale slowly through your nostrils.

    iv).   On completion breathe normally and relax.

5.1.7: 'HA' Sound cleansing Breathing.

This exercise is another version of cleansing breath that cleans and ventilates the lungs. It is also useful to practice this exercise after any other breathing exercises. It helps to increase mindfulness and the internal heat of the body.

How to practice

    i).   Stand straight with your feet together and your arms hanging loosely alongside your body.

    ii).   Take a deep breath and at the same time raise your arms overhead.

    iii).   Hold your breath for a few seconds then bend your body forward from your waist, lower your arms and expel the air from your mouth using a strong blast making a 'HA' sound

    iv).   The sound need not be forced but should be loud enough.

    v).   The forceful exhalation almost like a slight cough to empty the lungs completely.

    vi).   Repeat this exercise a few times.

    vii).   Stand straight, breath normally and relax.

CHAPTER SIX

Kumbhaka, (Breath Retention Techniques) of Pranayama

Breadth retention is the fundamental importance in Pranayama. Therefore, the retention technique must be learnt and understood properly to be able to practice Pranayama for its full benefits. The techniques of Pranayama relates to the whole area of psycho-physiology. When we inhale and retains the breath, the Prana in the body starts to distribute throughout the whole body which in effect decreases the energy in the body. By proper techniques of Pranayama, it helps to direct the Prana to those parts of the body where it is needed. There are two types of breathing. Namely, breathing through the lungs or external or outer breathing. By this method, it allows outer air to penetrate to the lungs by inhaling and exhaling.

The second types of breathing are the internal or cellular breathing. The primary object of Pranayama is to stimulate cells in the body which in turn increases the production of internal heat by the activation of intercellular combustion. Regular practice of proper Pranayama improves physiological dynamism, to improve the vital systems in the body and enables us to withstand all the stresses of life. The duration of breath holding and how it is used internally by will, depends on the proper controlled breathing, the Kumbhaka exercises. However, there are good effects as well as dangers of Kumbhaka. It is therefore, very important to know the duration of breadth retention and its effects in the body. Kumbhaka between 3-20 seconds is within everybody's reach and may be practised at any time. By this method of Kumbhaka, the oxygen absorption is increased than normal breathing at the same time carbon dioxide evacuation is more complete. Kumbhaka of 20-90 seconds creates much more pronounced reactions. It must be practiced under the guidance of a qualified instructor. Kumbhaka of ninety seconds and up to several minutes causes complete revitalisation in the body. It interrupts the oxygen supply in the lung and soon creates unfavourable conditions leading to asphyxia and eventually may lead to death if prolonged. During breath retention the carbon dioxide level in the blood raises and internal temperature tends to go up. Although breath retention stimulates body cells, and it increases Pranic exchanges in the whole body and these benefits may be gained without any danger provided we observe some basic rules. The respiratory mechanism of our body functions automatically works but it also works from the conscious self. The peculiarity of the respiratory system is that it can be controlled by conscious self for it to accelerate, slow them or even stop them. During Kumbhka, the conscious self gets the direct link with the respiratory centre and takes control of the whole mechanism of the respiratory system in the body and dictates the nervous system of the body. **However you should refrain from practice of Kumbhaka if you have heart problems.**

6.1: Basic cautionary rules of Kumbhaka (Breath retention:

Before practicing pranayama, empty your bladder, and, if possible, the bowels. Ideally, you should practice in the open air or in a well-ventilated room and if necessary in a heated room in the winter. It is advised to warm up the body for a few minutes by doing a few yoga asana before practicing Kumbhaka. Asana helps to increase the circulation of blood flow through the body, opens up the capillaries and enables Prana released during breath retention. However, prolonged breath retention may cause Pranic disturbances if the body is not ready to receive Prana when body is not been limbered up by asana. Never practice during the initial phase of digestion. It is advisable to wait at least 2-3 hours after food or longer before practicing prolonged retention of breath. Do not over practice if you get tired. If you feel very tired, stop practicing and take up Savasana,(The pose of tranquillity or the dead posture to relax.)

Savasana (The pose of tranquillity, the dead posture)

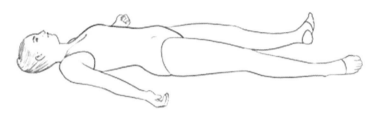

Figure 12

This posture is the best exercise for the complete relaxation of nerves, muscles and the mind quickly. Properly practiced this posture will reduce tension of the mind, anxiety, insomnia, and stress. This also helps to keep the blood pressure normal and improves vitality of the body and mind. Practising this posture properly for ten minutes is as good as sleeping for 3 hours. You should always finish your yoga by doing this exercise at the end. This exercise establishes muscular equilibrium quickly. The complete relaxation of all voluntary muscles is transferred to involuntary parts and produces the necessary equilibrium for the renewal of mental strength in a short period of time. Even more than sleep, successful relaxation is the vital principle of rest which quickly recuperates the nerve centres collects the scattered forces and reinvigorates the whole body. In partial relaxation, the attention should be practiced in following sequence: first the tips of the toes, then, slowly moving upwards, the ankles; the knees; the thighs; the anus; the generative organs; the navel the stomach; the heart; the neck; the lips; the tip of the nose; the eyes; the space between the eye brows; the forehead and finally the brain.

Stebbins observes that "Relaxation means the conscious transfer of energy from one department of nature to another, with perfect ease and grace, after an extreme tension of body or brain. True relaxation would mean a complete resignation of the body to the laws of gravity, the mind to nature, and the entire energy transferred to a deep dynamic breathing. The complete relaxation of the voluntary muscles at once transfers the energy to the involuntary parts, so that, strictly speaking, there can be no such thing as relaxation, except in the voluntary muscles and brain. But this is quite sufficient. This transfer of energy by voluntary action and involuntary reason produces the necessary equilibrium for the renewal of strength."

6.2: How to Practice

i).   i). Lie flat on your back with your arms alongside your body and palms facing upwards in complete relaxation.

ii).   Keep your legs straight and slightly apart

iii).   Keep your body completely motionless like a corpse and relax every muscle in your body gradually.

iv).   Close your eyes and place your attention first to the tips of your toes and then slowly moving upwards to the ankles, the knees, the thighs, the hips, the naval, the stomach, the heart, the neck, the tip of the nose, the eyes, the space between the eyebrows, the foreheads and finally the brain.

v).   Try to relax one part after another- all in this sequence as mentioned above. The best way to relax is to increase the tension first of these parts and release the tension consciously and completely switching off your attention from these parts.

6.3: Warming up process

Before beginning any asana or pranayama it is important to warm up the inner systems of our body by practicing a few exercises designed to warm up the body, loosen the muscles and joints, reduce stiffness, improve blood circulation and the body will be able to take up any undue stress or strain. It is always better to warm up your whole body from head to toe. There are several exercises as well as yoga exercises to warm-up your body and reduce stiffness of joints and muscles quickly. To prepare for exercises and to warm up and loosen your joints from head to toe are mentioned below in chapter seven.

CHAPTER SEVEN

7.1: Preparing for exercise

Before beginning the exercise, it is advisable to evacuate the bladder and bowel, clean the nose and the throat of all mucus and drink a glass of water.

Dress: Temperature and season permitting, open-air exercise is the best, whenever possible. In the case of indoor practice, however the room should be well ventilated but free from draughts kept at suitable angles.

The body should be free to move without any restriction. Clothing should always be loose, light and comfortable. In the floor: The floor exercises should be done on a rug, yoga mat or folded blankets or on a sleeping bag. The object is to ensure hygienic security, comfort and uniformity of temperature by insulating against very cold atmosphere.

7.2: General advice:

i).   Be sure that you have medical approval before embarking on physical yoga and pranayama. Make sure that there is nothing to forbid you doing certain inverted positions such as:

Headstand, Shoulder stand, Rapid abdominal breathing etc. as it may cause undesirable effects if you have heart disease or very high blood pressure or problems with eye or ear infections. Omit **Sun salutation (figure17a,b,c,d,f)**, if you are suffering from varicose veins.

ii). Do not practices yoga on a full stomach and after a heavy meal. Postures or asana and pranayama where excessive stomach contraction is needed should only be done on a complete empty stomach.

iii). Try to do the exercises at about the same time and same place every day or on a regular basis preferably in the morning in a convenient and quiet place for mind and body to be easily adaptable in anticipating further exercise.

iv). Always begin with the simplest exercise and slowly progress through more difficult ones.
v).   Always try to keep your mind away from other destructions. Concentrate on the exercises you are doing and the benefits you are gaining from each exercise.
vi). Before starting the exercise sit still for a few minutes preferably closing your eyes followed by a few cycles of deep breathing. Relax and let go all stiffness of your arms, legs and shoulders etc.

vii). vii). Always begin with a few warm-up exercises so that the body is ready to take any stress and strain of the exercises to follow.

viii). It is important to follow the instructions of the book carefully. A mis-reading or misunderstanding of an instruction could cause injury, and you should remember that nothing should ever be forced or strained. If you feel any excessive tension, stiffness or pain while doing any of the postures, you must stop at once and rest.

ix). Always finish your yoga exercise with the Pose of tranquillity (see Chapter 6, figure 12 and how to practice).

x). Expert advice and instructions are given at each step of the exercise for the maximum benefit. However, whatever asana you practice, remember that this time is your time, dedicated to yourself, your health, beauty, happiness and your peace of mind. The exact number of exercises and their duration is difficult to fix. But it should not be so meagre as to be ineffective. A half an hour a day is strongly recommended.

What needs to be emphasised, however, is that when for some reason or other the daily practice of yoga is missed, the same should be made good as soon as possible. This will maintain the daily health rhythm consequent upon the whole some equilibrium of a well-rounded hygienic life.

7.3: General exercise for the neck.

This exercise helps to reduce stiffness and enhance flexibility of the neck. This exercise can be done while sitting or standing.

i). Sit comfortably in a cross-legged position, body totally relaxed and breathe normally.

ii). Close your eyes, slowly bend your head forward so that your chin touches your chest and then backward as far as it can go without strain.

iii). Slowly lift your head straight and back to the starting position.

iv). Do this exercise only three times and look straight.

v). Close your eyes and slowly turn your neck to the left and then to the right as far as it can go without any strain.

vi). Do this exercise three times then look straight.

vii). Bend your head sideways on top of your shoulder to the left and right and straighten your head.

viii). Bend your head forward so that your chin touches your chest then turn your head clockwise over your left shoulder, at the back, over your right shoulder and back to the starting position.

ix). Repeat your exercise anti-clockwise and lift your head straight. Lift your shoulder up near your ear and relax.

7.4: Shoulder to Ear exercise.

This exercise will help to reduce tension around the shoulder and loosen up the muscles and joints around the neck and shoulder.

i). Sit comfortably on a cross-legged position or stand with your spine straight. Relax your face, shoulder, arms and hands.

ii). Lift your shoulders near your ears, turn them back squeezing your shoulder blades then down like a circular motion and relax.

iii). Bend your shoulder back squeezing your shoulder blades together, then lift your shoulders towards your ear, then forward and down in a circular motion in opposite direction. Relax your shoulders and breathe normally.

7.5: Warming up the upper body

The following exercises are designed to warm up the body fully to start practice of pranayama.

i). Stand straight with your arms alongside your body. Inhale and slowly lift your one arm straight over your head at the same time lift your body on your toes.

ii). Exhale, and at the same time lower your arm back to the original position. Lower your heels flat on the ground. Repeat this exercise a few times. Then repeat the same exercise with other arm a few times and relax.

iii). Stand straight with your arms alongside your body. Inhale and slowly lift your arms in line with your shoulder and inhale at the same time.

iv). Slowly lower your arms alongside your body and exhale. Repeat this exercise a few times and relax.

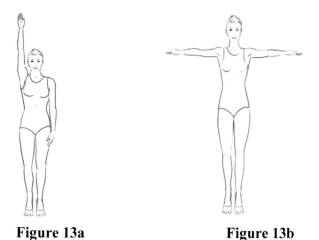

Figure 13a   Figure 13b

7.6: Forward bending

This exercise will bring lots of blood in the upper part of the body and loosen the hip joints.

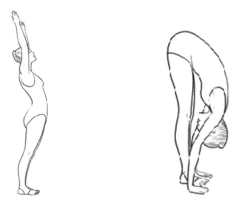

Figure 14a   Figure 14b

i). Stand straight with your arms alongside your body. Inhale and lift your arms over your head and clap your thumbs together, palm facing forward and your head between your arms.

ii). Exhale and slowly lower your body from your hip and touch the ground with your palms keeping your legs straight and your feet flat on the ground.

iii). Stay in this position for a while, then, inhale and while inhaling lift your body straight with your arms overhead and bend backward as far as back you can go still keeping your feet flat on the ground.

iv). Exhale and while exhaling, straighten your body, lower your arms sideways back to the original position and relax.

7.7: Squatting

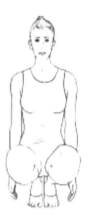

Figure 15

This exercise will stretch the muscles around your thigh and legs and loosen your knee and ankle joints. This also helps to restore body balance.

i). Stand straight, lift your arms forward and parallel to the ground.

ii). Slowly, lower your body bending your knees still keeping your arms straight and your heels flat on the ground.

iii). When you cannot go down any further, lift your body on your toes and squat on your heels. Lower your arms on your knees.

iv). Stay in this position for a while then lift your arm again parallel to the ground. Lift your body very slowly straighten your toes without bending forward. Lower your heels flat on the ground and your arms alongside your body and relax.

7.8: Warming up lower part of the body (The lying twist:

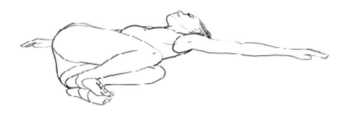

Figure 16a

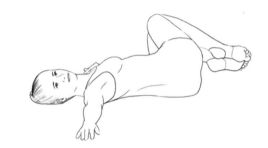

Figure 16b

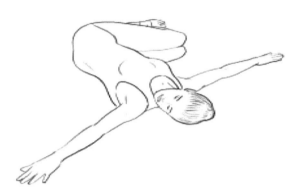

Figure 16c

This exercise warms up the lower parts of the body particularly the abdominal and the pelvic region. It strengthens the abdominal muscles and the lower back and increases the flexibility of the pelvic region.

As shown in the figures16a, 16b, and 16c, do the exercises as follows:

  i).   Lie on your back with yours arms stretched in line with your shoulder and the legs straight with your toes together.
  ii).   Bend your knees closer to your body so that your heels are flat on the ground.
  iii). Inhale and lift your knees and bring them closer to your chest keeping your toes together.
  iv).   Exhale and while exhaling keeping your shoulder, arms and back of your head in contact with the ground slowly and smoothly tilt and bend your knees on one side trying to touch the ground on that side.
  v).   Inhale and bring your knees back to the upright position near your chest.
  vi).   Exhale and bend your knees back to the opposite side still keeping your head shoulder and arms flat on the ground.
  vii). Inhale and bring your knees back to the upright position and repeat this exercise a few times.

viii). On completion, stretch your legs straight and relax.

7.9: Surya Namaskar (The Sun Salutation:

This is a complete exercise for the body muscles, joints and the circulatory process of the body. This exercise warms up the body by increasing the blood circulation and later cools down the body to restore the normal state. It helps to develop concentration, relieves tensions of the mind and reduces stress. It is very useful exercise for the lymphatic system to eliminate the waste matters from the body and develops the immune system of the body. You should practice this exercise in proper sequence as mentioned below with particular attention to the breathing sequence. Do not practice this exercise if you are suffering from high blood pressure, varicose veins or hernia.

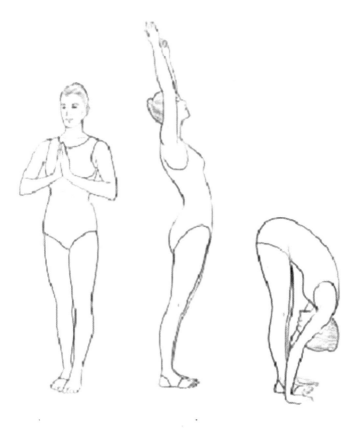

Figure 17a   **Figure 17b**   **Figure 17c**

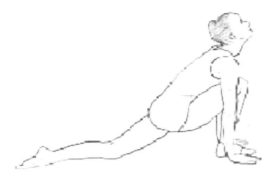

Figure 17d

34

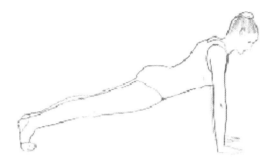

Figure 17e

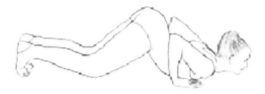

Figure 17f

7.9.1: How to practice

i).   Stand straight with your toes and heels together and bring your palms together near your body similar to the prayer posture and breathe normally.

ii). Inhale and raise your arms straight over your head and bend your body backwards as far back as you can go keeping your heels flat on the ground.

iii). Exhale and bend forward keeping your head between your arms and place your hands on the ground on both sides of your feet.

iv). Inhale and lift your head up and breathe normally. Stay in this position for a while.

v).   Inhale again and while holding your breath shift your left leg back and lower your left knee on the ground at the same time bend your right knee so that thigh touches the right chest still keeping your palms on the ground.

vi). Straighten your left leg and lift your left knee above the ground. Stay in this position for a while and breathe normally.

vii). Slowly stretch your right leg in line with your left leg and keep your toes together. Taking the body weight on your palm lift both knees above the ground and continue to breathe normally.

viii). .Inhale and lower your body and knees on the ground and arch your back and lift your head up, and breathe normally.

ix). Lift your body and take the left leg forward bending from your knees so that the left thigh is touching the chest and straighten your right leg at the back and breathe normally.

x).   Follow the sequence as you did with your other leg to the cobra position.

xi). Inhale and take the body weight on your palm and lift your body from the ground. Slowly sit down on your heels and lift your body on your legs to the starting position and relax for a while in the standing position for your body to cool down.

xii). You can repeat the whole sequence of the series posture if you want.

7.10: Bidalasana (The Cat Stretch Series Posture:

This cat stretch series follows the sequence of postures the same way a cat tones up its body. These postures help to get cat like suppleness and the agility of the body. They increase the suppleness of the spine, reduce fat on the abdomen, and improve circulation of the whole body. They help to reduce constipation by improving the digestive systems.

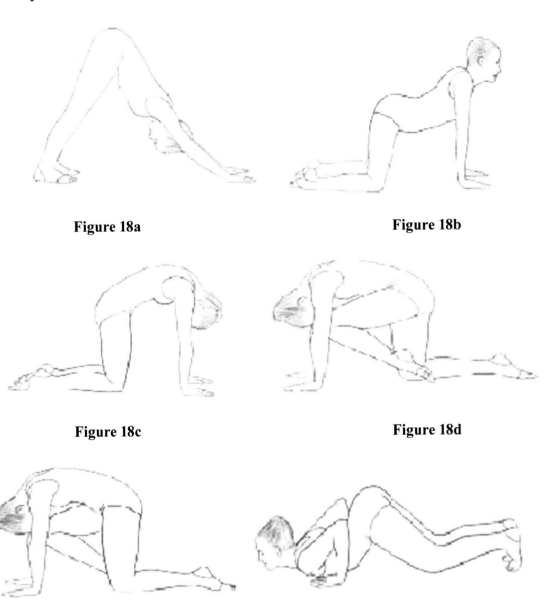

Figure 18a

Figure 18b

Figure 18c

Figure 18d

Figure 18e

Figure 18f

7.10.1: How to Practice

1. Support your body using your palms and knees on the ground, fingers of the palm pointing ahead. Keep your knees together and the palms about shoulder width apart.
2. Keep your toes together, legs straight in line with your body. Inhale and raise your head, straighten your elbow and thighs so that both hands and thighs are vertical to the ground and your back and head are parallel to the ground then exhale.
3. Inhale and lower your back between the shoulder and the hips as much as you can and lift your head high. Stay in this position for a while then exhale. Bring your back parallel to the ground and lower your head parallel to the ground.
4. Inhale, and then exhale at the same time. Lift your spine upward like a hump as high as you can and bring your head between yours arms.
5. Stay in this position for a while then inhale and lower your back between the shoulders and hips as mentioned in instruction 3 and repeat the whole sequence a few times.
6. On completion, support your body as mentioned in instruction 1.
7. Take the weight of the body on your palms. Shift the right leg straight with knees on the ground, and then lift your left leg so that left knee is closer to your chest and feet flat on the ground. Lift your right knee above the ground and breathe normally.
8. Stay in this position for a while then stretch your left leg straight and bring your right knee near the body, same as instruction 7 but with other leg.
9. On completion, stretches both legs straight and lower it flat from your knee to toe on the ground. At the same time, bend your elbow up and resume the Cobra position mentioned earlier with your hips and head above the ground.
10. Slowly lift your body from the ground taking the weight on your palms. At the same time bend your knees one at a time and resume the standing position.
11. Bend your right leg and bring the right knee between your arms taking the body weight on both arms and the left knee. Keep your left leg flat on the ground from knee to the toe and the head lowered between your arms.
12. Repeat the exercise as mentioned in instruction 11 with your other leg.
13. On completion resume the starting position.
14. Inhale and lift your right leg and straighten it in line with your body. Lift your head and exhale.
15. Repeat the exercise mentioned in instruction 14 with the other leg.
16. Resume the starting position and relax.

7.11: Precaution before practicing Pranayama

Before practicing pranayama close your eye or concentrate at the tip of your nose and place your tongue at the top of the gums of upper front teeth or bend it back against the soft palate. If necessary swallow your saliva.

i). During Pranayama with Kumbhaka, the spine must be straight and vertical so that the weight of the body is distributed evenly with pelvic area slightly forwards for Pranic currents to run through the spinal column from lowest position to the brain. The anus must be contacted and raised. During inhalation, you should breathe slowly, uniformly and completely concentrating while closing the eyes during penetration of air through the nostril. The active participation of mind for concentration is also very important to get the maximum benefit.

ii). It should not be performed lying down except some breathing exercises can be practiced while lying down in the Savasana posture or in the bed.

iii). Breath retention must only be performed on an empty stomach or at least one and half to five hours after the last meal.

iv). For Kumbhaka practice, sit down either in the **Lotus (Padmasana),** Vajrasana (**Diamond posture)** as shown in figure 19a and 19b) in order to slowdown the circulation in the legs to the benefit of heart and brain.

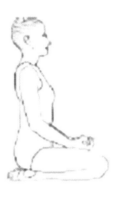

Diamond posture
Figure 19a

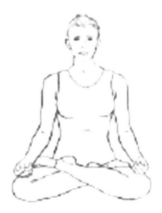

Lotus posture
Figure 19b

v). Deep, slow and complete breathing should be practiced before breadth retention except before Kapalbhati and Bhastica. Concentration is also essential avoiding all distractions to gain the maximum benefit while practicing Pranayama, where deep, slow and complete breathing cause a massive expulsion of carbon dioxide in the body, and, it is needed to direct the carbon dioxide for the chemical aquarium of the blood. During retention, the heartbeats slow down to a calm but stronger rhythm, though it varies from person to person depending on body's demand. At the same time, the exhalation too must be slow, smooth, gradual and continuous but the last trace of air should be exhaled with force by contracting the rib-cage and abdomen and wait for one or two seconds for the inhalation to start again. If you hold your breath and begin to feel that you about to burst then you have exceeded your capabilities. In that case, reduce the length of retention.

vi). Beginners should always remember that just holding the breath in the lung for a long time not necessarily mean that you will get all the benefits of pranayama immediately. Therefore, length and frequency of retention should be increased very gradually. To hold the breath correctly you must take at least five complete and deep breaths. Extend the practice of breath retention gradually until you feel a sensation of fatigue, but, not when you feel suffocated.

vii). **Jalandhara Bandha** may be practiced in all stages of respiratory acts of pranayama. Jalandhara bandha is a technique to hold the breath properly (in long retention) when the lung is full with inhalation. The methods of this bandha is to hold your breath and swallow your saliva then contract your throat muscles, then place your chin in the fork of the sternum. It is important to place the chin at this precise spot to block and seal the breath of the chest and prevents the air to come up to nostril and it is impossible to breath. While practicing pranayama, it is essential to avoid development of air pressure beyond glottis (entrance to the wind pipe). Although, it is possible to block the breath, without bending the throat and glottis and it is perfectly safe and possible to retain the breath for short retentions. For long retention, it is important to use Jalandara technique which acts gently on the nerves and in turn acts as a safety lock to retain the breath in the chest. It serves to protect the heart and the vascular system from ill effects of prolonged breath retention.

It is very useful to practice and Halasana (plough postures, figure 20a) Sarvangasan (the shoulder stand, figure 20b) before using Jalandhara Bandha. However, If you have high blood pressure, then, you should avoid these asana.

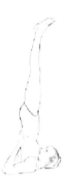

Halasana (Plough posture)
Figure 20a

Sarvangasan (Shoulder stand))
Figure 20b

In practicing pranayama, the rhythm of the breathing is also very important. The most important rhythms are those of the heart. The rhythm of our heart beats depends on the power of our heart muscles. For example, the blood flow in our body depends on our physiological needs. The heart beats of a running man is faster and accelerates if we increase the speed of running compared to a person's heart beat requirements when resting. As we generally know, in normal breathing we inhale and exhale 16-20 per minute, hearts beats from 72-80 per minute and our one respiration delivers sufficient oxygen to do all that. Rhythm also affects our endurance. Therefore, it is possible and important to control the rhythm of the body at will. Our physiological and psychological functions of the body can be deliberately controlled by altering rhythmic pattern of our breathing. To get the right rhythmic breathing, you need to take time for you to get the normal resting breathing when you can concentrate your heartbeats by taking your pulse at the wrist at the same time try to synchronise the respiratory rhythms consciously by counting 2 beats for inhaling, four for exhaling and breathe for about one minute. Normally, our rhythm breathing for exhalation lasts twice as long as inhalation. To obtain best benefit of rhythm breathing, gradually lengthen the count of inhalation of count of three heart beats, six for exhalation. When you find this breathing is without any discomfort or effort, increase to four beats for inhalation and eight beats for exhalation. You will soon find that you have developed perfect synchronisation. There are two types of rhythmic breathing namely: Complete rhythmic breathing and alternate rhythmic breathing. In complete rhythmic breathing, you need to inhale for one unit, followed by four units of Kumbhaka and exhalation for two units (ratio of 1:4:2). In other words, the inhalation for four heart beats (1 unit), holding the breath with full lungs for sixteen heart beats (16 heart beats (4units) and exhale for eight heart beats (2 units). The alternate rhythmic breathing should be practiced when you have become accustomed to the rhythmic breathing technique. It is important not to rush through any stages.

At the end of pranayama session relax for a few minutes using Savasana (Dead posture as shown in figure 12). This exercise is made up of four stages and performed lying flat on the back on some hard surface with arms by the sides of the body. Then consciously relax the muscles of the body concentrating from the tips of the toes upwards, relaxing feet, ankles, calves, knees, thighs, abdominal muscles, chest and shoulders arms and hands, finally facial muscles. Then close your eyes and try to wipe out any tension of the forehead. In other words, every single muscle should be relaxed so as to feel limp and lifeless inducing a feeling of letting go, literally as if you cannot even raise your hands. Switch off all thoughts and try to keep your mind blank as long as you can. Initially it will be difficult to relax properly, but, with practice you find that you will find yourself refreshed as if you had several hours of sleep. From regular practice you will gain benefits if you are suffering from tension, insomnia, nervous disorder, and high blood-pressure or heart conditions.

CHAPTER EIGHT

8.1: Types of Pranayama & their benefits

There are several very simple and also difficult ways to practice pranayama. You should practice which are most suitable and beneficial for you. During pranayama, the lungs hold both oxygen and Prana. There are different breathing techniques of pranayama, especially using strong intra-abdominal pressure which improves the function of the heart. It is important to learn and understand how and when to use abdominal muscle control. However, muscle control is not necessarily synonymous with contraction of abdomen. For each type of pranayama, there is a specific way to breath and control of breathing, using lung and abdominal muscles.

8.2: Simple Deep Breathing Pranayama.

This pranayama is very simple to practice but have many advantages. It may be practiced in a yoga posture or in a low chair, lying down in the bed before falling asleep, or in the morning before getting up, and also while walking except when there are smog, or dust in the air while walking. This pranayama may also be practiced where number of stages and cycles can vary at will and is very comfortable without any pressure and with many benefits. In this exercise, rhythm plays an essential part. Method of this pranayama is very simple. Just breathe in counting 1,2,3,4 or more with one or both nostrils until the lung is full. Then exhale through your mouth, counting the same number of breathing time. In other words, the timing of both inhaling and exhaling are the same. You then follow the normal breathing. You may practice this pranayama for 20 to 30 times with or without break.

By this Pranayama, our lung receives more oxygen by forced breathing than normal breathing. The benefits of this pranayama are inhaling more oxygen in the lung, which expands the diaphragm and improves the metabolism in the body. It also helps our digestive system.

Since this pranayama can be practiced while walking, it is advisable not to practice this pranayama where there are dust or exhaust from cars on the street.

8.3: Delayed Exhale Pranayama.

This pranayama is the same as the deep breathing pranayama except the time of exhaling is twice the time of inhaling. In other words, inhale counting 1,2,3,4 or more to fill the lung. Then exhale at the double the timing (4x2) of inhaling time. In other words Inhale counting 1,2,3,4 or more to fill the lung then exhale counting 1 to 8, taking double time of inhaling.

In this pranayama, by exhaling the breadth is twice longer than breathing time, you are exhaling more carbon dioxide. By this pranayama, it helps to increase the functions of both the heart and the lung. This pranayama is very useful for those who have high blood pressure or have weak heart function.

8.4: Pranayama while lying down

This pranayama is practiced while lying down. It is very useful for those who have weak health or those who gets tired very easily. To get the benefit of this pranayama, you need to lie down in 'Savasana posture'. (As shown in figure 12). While lying down, you may use both deep breathing or delayed exhale pranayama. In addition, while breathing, lift your arms over your head and touch the ground on the sides of your head then while exhaling bring your arms by the side of your body. You may also perform this pranayama by using one hand at a time. This pranayama have the same benefits of deep breathing and delayed exhale breathing.

8.5: Pranayama while walking.

This pranayama is practiced while walking. Breathe, while walking and counting 1,2,3,4,5,6... or more of each step of walking, then exhale in one and half or twice the time of inhaling count. You can practice initially for 5-10 minutes and gradually increase the timing up to 30 minutes.

This pranayama is very useful mainly for old people or those who cannot practice any other pranayama in a sitting posture.

8.6: Sitkari Pranayama.(Hissing breath:

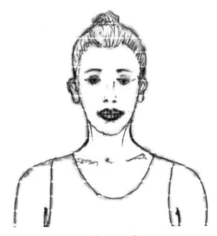

Figure 21

This pranayama is practiced simply breathe through the gaps in the teeth. In Sanskrit, Sitkari means "hissing sound. In Sitkari pranayama, while breathing through gaps of the teeth, a "hiss" sound is produced.. Breathe in through the gaps of the teeth to fill the lung and exhale through the nostril as shown in figure 21.

To practice Sitkari sit on an Easy pose or Lotus posture. Gently press the upper and lower teeth together then inhale through the gaps of the teeth filling the abdomen and exhale through the nose closing your lips

By this pranayama, both the heart and lung increase their functions. This pranayama especially useful for those who have high blood pressure. It helps to reduce anxiety, hypertension, hyper acidity, calms down the mind and improves the good health of the teeth.

8.7: Sitali Pranayama. (Cooling breath:

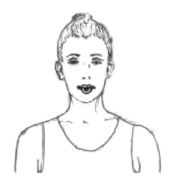

Figure 22

This pranayama is a minor exercise, especially useful in hot weather where atmosphere air temperature is high. This pranayama is practiced by breathing through the mouth and also exhaling through the nostril. Make your mouth opening round and small and breathe in to fill your lungs then retain the breath for 5 seconds then slowly breathe out through your nostril. This pranayama is very useful to cool down the inner heat of the lung, like an air cooler machine. This is very useful in hot climate and for those who are suffering from high blood pressure.

Note: Both Sitkari and Sitali pranayama yoga removes excess heat from the inner body and keeps the body temperature down, relaxes nerves, brain, cures insomnia, stress, controls hunger and thirst, removes acidity and also prevents premature greying and hair fall.

8.8: Vilom Pranayama, (method using fractional inhalation:.

This pranayama may be performed either in yoga posture or in a low chair, may also be performed while walking or even lying down. To practice this pranayama, follow these methods:

a. first determine the rhythm of your heart beats.
b. then inhale through both nostrils for two heart beats,
c. hold your breath for two heart beats,
d. inhale again for two heart beats
e. stop your breath again for two heart beats
f. hold your breath for five-ten seconds, and exhale slowly through both nostrils. When the lungs are empty, repeat the same process again for five times followed by fractional exhalation.

8.9: Vilom Pranayama, method using fractional exhalation

The exhalation is performed in successive stages. Just two beats for retention, two beats for exhalation, two beats for retention and two beats exhalation and so on until lungs are quite empty. After a retention for five to ten seconds, inhale without any interruption. The fractional inhalation and exhalation may be repeated several times provided you do not feel tired. When there is a feeling of fatigue or discomfort, you must stop Pranayama. Increasing the duration is not necessarily beneficial when you are tired.

When both fractional inhalation and exhalation becomes very familiar, it is advisable to get further benefit, if you do the Mula Bandha (by contracting the anal muscles while retention for both fractional inhalation and fractional exhalation) at the same time. During Mula Bandha you should concentrate on the anal area. If you have heart problem, then you should refrain from Mula Bandha. It has the special advantage of normalising for people suffering from both high and low blood pressure.

8.10: The Pranayama square:

This pranayama exercise has four phases, inhalation, retention, exhalation and retention, where all stages are of the same duration. Begin by exhaling the lung and hold your lung when empty for the count of 1,2,3,4,or more then inhale counting same numbers 1,2,3,4,…, or more then retain with full lung for the same count of 1,2,3,4,…or more then empty your lung counting same numbers1,2,3,4…more. Repeat the cycle as many times as you can confidently practice without resting in between depending on the capacity of your lungs. You may increase the count more than four times depending on the capacity of your lungs. This pranayama trains the lungs for prolonged retention without any danger or side effects

This pranayama includes, rhythm, mental concentration, breath retention and control of vital processes. This pranayama can be practiced by all without any fear or danger of side effects or discomfort. This pranayama prepares the whole body for an increased pranic circulation and allow a better revitalisation of the human being.

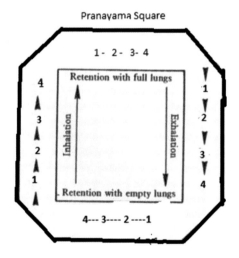

Pranayama square Figure 23

8.11: Anulom & Bilom Pranayama.

This Pranayama is involves inhaling and exhaling with retention of breath. Anulom and Bilom is a very important and classical Pranayama exercise. For methods of Kumbhaka, read Chapter Six before attempting.

As mentioned in Chapter Six, Kumbhaka between 3-20 seconds is within everybody's reach and may be practised at any time. By this method of Kumbhaka, the oxygen absorption is increased than normal breathing at the same time carbon dioxide evacuation is more complete. Kumbhaka of 20-90 seconds creates much more pronounced reactions and it is advised to practice under the guidance of a qualified instructor. If the retention stage lasts for more than 10 seconds then Jalandhara Bandha becomes obligatory. According to old scriptures, 'Jala' means 'nerves which passes through the neck towards the brain'. From the yogic point of view, the purpose of Bandha means is to bind or to awaken and control the subtle Pranic energy present in our bodies.

According to quote from 'Shiva Samhita' scripture, the explanation of Jala Bandha expressed as: "The chin is pressed against the triangular hollow formed at the junction of collar bones and this causes pressure on the Centre of Extreme Purity situated in the neck. When properly done, this contraction blocks the respiratory apparatus and, when the breath is held (Kumbhaka), it prevents the nerve which passes through the neck towards the brain".

It is essential to place the chin correctly at this precise spot in order to achieve one of the main objectives of Jalandhara and must always accompany any prolonged breath retention. The main purpose of Jalandhara is to compress the throat, to contract the neck muscle, and stretching the cervical vertebrae to contract and seals the neck muscles during the whole of Jalandhara Bandha and prevent breathing.

The Anuloma and Biloma exercise may be practiced as follows:

Exhale through the left nostril; Inhale through the left nostril; Kumbhaka with full lungs (initially between 3-20 seconds); Exhale through the right nostril; Inhale through the right nostril; Kumbhaka with full lungs. Devote this cycle for at least five minutes strictly following the rules of Kumbhaka.

8.12: Bhastrika, the Bellows Pranayama

The Bhastika has taken its name from bellows of blacksmith. As mentioned in old scriptures, Bhastrika: "As the Blacksmith's bellows dilate and contract continuously, so the yogi inhales slowly through the nostrils while distending the abdomen; he/she expels the air rapidly (when it makes the same noise as bellows)".

This pranayama should be practiced by the control of abdominal belt in Siddhasana and Lotus postures (as shown in figures 7 and 9). Simply breathe slowly to fill the lung and exhale the air rapidly for 10-20 times. Then inhale and perform Kumbhaka (retention of breath) for a few seconds then exhale rapidly with force. While practicing this pranayama, during the whole exercise, the spine should be straight and immobile. While, practicing, nostril should be absolutely free. This pranayama helps to saturate the oxygen in the blood by expelling a large quantity of carbon dioxide which in turn a considerable acceleration of blood flow goes in the brain. Hence, it must be done without violence. By practicing progressively, the lungs will become more elastic for maximum benefit.

8.13: Kapalbhati Pranayama

The name Kapalbhati came from the Sanskrit root. Kapal means the skull and Bhati means to clean. It literally means 'cleaning the skull. Where skull includes, the nostril, the ears, and other air ducts inside the skull. In this pranayama, breathing is slow and passive where exhalation is active and forceful.

This exercise can be practiced in Siddhasan, Vajrasan or sitting in the lotus posture.(As shown in figure 9b). While practicing this pranayama, your spine should be strait, and the chest should be blocked with full of air. Then you need to contract the muscle of the abdomen sharply to expel the air violently with force. Then slowly relax the abdomen so as to protrude the abdomen while inhaling slowly and silently with progressive relaxation of the abdomen. The function and control of the abdomen is the main requirement while breathing both in and out. You may increase the speed gradually first say 10-40 exhalations per minute and then to maximum of 120 per minute. The inhalation should be at least three times longer than exhalation.

It is also useful to practice Kapalbhati even before the beginning of asana. That will get rid of all the air remaining in the lungs and to ensure a good oxygenation of the blood.

The practice of Kapalbhati is helpful to clean the lungs. Substantial expulsion of carbon dioxide takes place from the blood and gets saturated with oxygen. Kapalbhati is an incomparable tonic for the entire nervous system of the body. However, it is advisable to get proper supervision if you wish to do intensive practice.

Proper practice of Kapalbhati and the effects of inhalation of Kapalbhati exercise and its respiratory movement have a profound effect on the brain. The brain behaves like spongy mass, shrinking and enlarging according to the respiratory rhythm and influences the circulation of fluids in the brain and blood within the normal physiological limits. Hence the Kapalbhati exercise affects the 'brain washing' process. Hence, Kapalbhati pranayama stimulates the brain and its central nervous system and our thinking organ directly and acts as a pure and unique brain tonic and increases our powers of concentration, improves our memory and stimulates our intellectual faculties. This, the power of concentration, is the key to the treasure-house of knowledge. But, in our day to day life and in our present state of our body we are so much distracted, and the mind is flittering away its energies upon a hundred sorts of things. As soon as we try to calm our thoughts and concentrate our minds in any one object of knowledge, thousands of undesired impulses rush into our brains and thousands of thoughts rush into the mind and disturb it. How to check them and bring our mind under control is the essence of pranayama.

8.14:. Bhramari Pranayama

Bhramari pranayama technique includes making a humming sound like a bee using exhaling in a relaxed upright position. Bhramari pranayama breathing exercise has tremendous therapeutic potential. It effects the autonomic nervous system (ANS) of the body and activates the calming parasympathetic branch of the ANS.

8.14.1:.How to practice

Sit up straight on a lotus posture and place your hands on your face with one thumb on each ear blocking the ear passage. Close your eyes and place the index fingers on your fore head, the middle finger and the ring finger and little finger on your eyes lightly touching the eyes without any pressure on the eye balls. Breathe in through your nose. Make a buzzing sound through your lips of moderate volume on the exhalation as long as it's comfortable and you can still inhale smoothly, without gasping for air. Keep your facial muscles loose, your lips lightly touching, and your jaw relaxed, with the upper and lower rows of teeth slightly separated

When you make a sound, you will experience the vibration from the top of your head down to the tips of your toes. You may also make different pitches of vibration at different frequencies. Bass notes and other low-pitched sounds vibrate slowly, whereas high-pitched sounds vibrate quickly. Practice this exercise four to six times-

All though very few of the potential therapeutic applications of Bhramari have been studied scientifically, the yoga tradition teaches that well-chosen sounds have powerful and salutary effects for people suffering from Insomnia, Sinus infection or Nasal congestion, Thyroid problems and Stress. 8.15). Ujjayi Pranayama Ujjayi Pranayama is the process of deep inhaling and exhaling through both nostrils with a half closed glottis. The inhalation and exhalation process of this pranayama, a typical sound like the ocean is produced because of the friction of air within the throat. The sound is made completely different from the sound emitted from the larynx hence, the Pranayama is termed as "Ocean sound breath". The name derived from the Sanskrit word "Ujjayi" means to be victorious. This particular pranayama aims to keep the mind cool and the body warm. The inhalations and exhalations are of same duration. Ujjayi Pranayama helps to increase the action of oxygenation which helps to build internal body heat. Regular practice of this pranayama increases the blood circulation throughout the body and improves overall body metabolism. It also helps to eliminate accumulated toxins of the body and regulates blood pressure.

8.15.1: How to Practice

i).   it in any meditative posture like (Padmasana (Lotus pose) with eye closed and try to keep your spine erect. ii).Inhale slowly and deeply from both the nostril and try to contract the throat making sure the air is not touching the inside of the nose

ii).   Exhale slowly through your nose while constricting the muscles in the back of your throat.

iii). Feel the air passing through your wind pipe as you practise the process. (As air touches the throat a peculiar sound is produced.)

iv).   Contract the rear of your throat, making a gentle hissing sound as you inhale.

v).   Retain the breath for a while within full awareness without any strain (You may increase the retention when you are used to longer retention without any strain or discomfort).

vi).   Exhale making sure the sound isn't forced; but loud enough so if one can hear it sitting nearby.

vii). Then close your right nostril and exhale from the left nostril.

viii). Repeat the exercise for two or three cycles initially and increase it when you have mastered the technique.

Note: Refrain from practicing this pranayama if you are a patient of hypertension Make sure the proportion of the breathing is not forced while breathing

CHAPTER NINE

Mudras for Pranayama

There are many Mudras associated with the practice of Pranayama. In Sanskrit mudras means symbolic hand gestures primarily used during the practice of Pranayama. Mudras are considered as a part of a system where by energetic circuit passes through the network of 'Nadis' which enhances the flow of 'pranic' energy in the body.

There are several mudras used to practice Pranayama, and each Mudra has a specific benefit or a particular Pranayama. Foer example:

9.1:. Vishnu Mudra:

This mudra is used during Nadi Shodhana (To purify the nadis) while practicing Pranayama, when alter net breathing through nostrils are used such as Anulom Belom pranayama mentioned in Chapter 8.11.

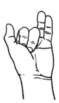

Figure 24

9.2:.Chin Mudra (Psychic gesture of consciousness::

In this mudra the hands rest on knees or thigh facing down. This gesture represents the classical (Gunas) or qualities of nature. The middle finger symbolises Sattva (purity, wisdom and understanding faculties), the ring finger symbolises Rajas (action, passion and movement of the body), whereas the little finger symbolises Tamas (inertia, lethargy and darkness). The main idea of these postures according to Yogis, is to transcend these states, progressing into light and from ignorance to wisdom.

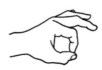

Figure 25

9.3:. Jnana Mudra (Psychic gesture of knowledge::

In this Mudra, the hands are placed on the knees with palms facing up while practicing Pranayama in sitting posture. This Mudra helps to uplift the effects of the body and mind. The connection made by thumb and index finger is said to create re-circulating the body's vital energy through Nadis.

Figure 26

9.4:. Chinmaya Mudra (Gesture of awareness::

In this Mudra the index finger and the thumb touches lightly while all other fingers are curls in the palm. This Mudra is said to influence the Prana in the thoracic area of the body.

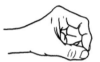

Figure 27

9.5:. Aadi Mudra (First gesture::

In this Mudra, the fingers are curled around the thumb making a very light fist. This Mudra positively influences the breathing and has a soothing influence on the mind. This Mudra helps to quieten the nervous system of the body especially while practicing Savasana at the end of Asana practice.

Figure 28

9.6:. Bramha Mudra (Gesture of all pervading consciousness::

In this Mudra, all fingers are wrapped around the thumbs and the knuckles of both and are pressed tightly together. This Mudra helps to stimulate a full breath in pranayama practice.

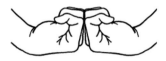

Figure 29

CHAPTER TEN

10.1: Cooling down exercises

According to ancient yogis, relaxation after Pranayama yoga gives maximum amount of renewed strength in the minimum amount of time. Even more than sleep, successful relaxation is the vital principle of rest which quickly recuperates or galvanises the neve centres, collects the scattered forces and reinvigorates the whole body. As warming up the body is important before starting any pranayama yoga exercises, cooling down your body is equally important to normalise the internal system. While practicing pranayama yoga all the internal systems such as, circulatory system, respiratory system, endocrine system, digestive system and nervous system start to function, similarly cooling down after the exercise is also very important to help prevent sudden drop in blood pressure that may cause dizziness or even fainting. It is therefore advised to take sufficient time to relax after practicing pranayama. The pose of tranquillity (dead posture, figure 12) in chapter six is recommended by the yoga authorities. In this case of concentration through relaxation will have the maximum benefit to cool down the whole body and mind..

The relaxation should not be mistaken for inertia; it also does not mean lying in a lazy manner or doing nothing You should withdraw all the voluntary nerve-force from the extremities and thinking part of the brain by concentration on the incoming and outgoing breath, however, the supply of nervous stimuli is switched off from all parts of the body simultaneously instead by stages. It is also important when relaxing the muscles is that the consciousness of the physical body should be necessarily and entirely forgotten.

It is best to practice relaxation in solitude with a view to ensure privacy and quietude. Then, with perfect silence through that listening attitude, which is directed towards the mind to abstraction by allowing respiratory acts to pass beyond conscious effort. In the case of concentration through relaxation, the synchronous void of abstraction devoid of sensorial impression should be utilised to identify oneself mentally with the object of concentration.

The pose of tranquillity mentioned as shown in figure 12 is the best cooling down exercise to cool the body quickly. Abruptly stopping after exercise without cooling your system may cause damage to your system.

The crocodile posture or Makarasana may also be very useful to cooldown your body. Makarasana has the similar benefits to the pose of tranquillity but it is performed differently. This relaxation technique can be used any time even on the bed. However, the bed should have a hard mattress without any pillow.

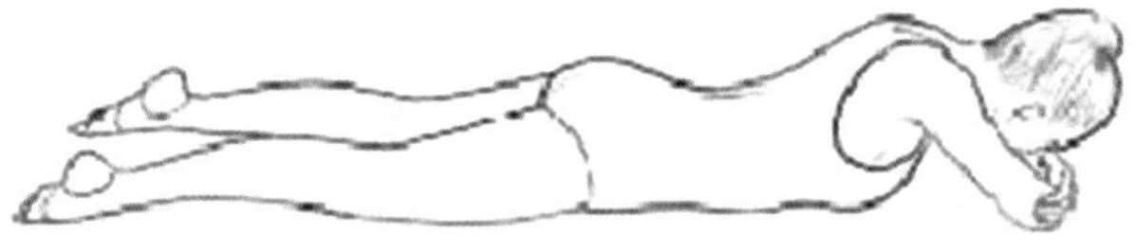

Makarasana (The Crocodile Posture)
Figure-30

10.2: How to Practice

1. Lie flat on your abdomen with legs fully stretched, toes pointed inward and separated.
2. Fold your arms so that one palm is on top of the other and rest your head on one side on top of your palms.
3. Close your eyes and breathe slowly and rhythmically. Concentrate your attention from your toes to your head and relax each part consciously similar to the pose of tranquillity
4. After a while change your head to other side and continue with the rhythmic breathing.

Conclusion

Appraisal and research of the Scientific Investigations of Pranayama it was found that virtually all the functions of the body are influenced by it. By regular practice of Pranayama the body becomes supple and the digestive and metabolic functions of the body become very efficient. Regular practice of Pranayama one feels extremely energetic, the need of the sleep becomes less. Practice of Pranayama also affects the mind, increases the power of concentration, and stabilizes the emotional effects of the mind.

By scientific observation of Pranayama, it was established; when we breathe there is a movement of our chest and thoracic diaphragm. These movements are always interdependent. Ordinarily it is not easy to move them independently or separately. But through the practice of Pranayama by using some specific technique one can learn to do so. This increases the ability to use the muscles of the chest and thoracic diaphragm in an independent way as is necessary.

In our normal breathing, the pressure inside the cavity of the chest and the abdomen increases or decreases during the process of exhalation and inhalation. In the practice of Kumbhaka of Pranayama, the pressure in the lungs changes and becomes more intense, resulting in vigorous massage of the various internal organs. It also enhances the blood circulation inside these organs, which stimulates their functions, and by exciting the nerve endings lying in the pleural lining of the chest and peritoneal lining of the abdominal cavity, as well as those inside our internal organs.

During the practice of Pranayama, it helps to increase our ability to maintain Kumbhaka for a long time, and, it prevents any adverse effects on the very delicate organs like lungs, heart, liver etc. It was also established by medical experiment that the ventilation of the breathing action, the air moves continuously in and out of the lungs when the breath is deep but very slow. At the same time as more amount of air taken in, and as it remains inside for a long time, the exchange of oxygen and carbon-dioxide inside the lungs is not much affected. However in the practice of Kapalbhati or the first part of the Bhastrika Pranayama, the breathing is very fast, the number of breaths in one minute is remarkably high and even though each breath is shallower than the normal breath. The minute ventilation as well as the effective alveolar ventilation show marked increase. As a result, the gaseous exchange is affected to some extent in the form of more extraction of carbon-dioxide from the blood into the alveolar air. The absorption of oxygen in the blood which even in normal breathing is around 92% to 96% of the saturation level, cannot be increased further and therefore does not show any change. Thus carbon-dioxide washout the main effect of this fast breathing variety of Pranayama, but when compared to the same effect as in hyper-ventilation it is still much less and does not lead to any imbalance in the acidity or alkalinity of the blood. This is because ordinarily when one holds the breath, the CO_2 level in the blood slowly starts rising up and when it goes beyond certain critical level, one has to start a process of breathing out to remove this CO_2. But, if the CO_2 level is already low after Kapalbhati, one can retain the breath much longer till CO_2 level in the blood could reach that critical level.

The scientific study also shows, the effect of Pranayama, on the functions of the heart, it has been observed that the blood pressure increases slightly in Kapalbhati and in Bhastrika Pranayama. Through the specific techniques of Pranayama, especially the one involving Kumbhaka for a long time, it is observed that one is able to gain a voluntary control over many of these visceral functions. It is recorded that one is able to reduce the heart rate or alter the circulation of blood in different regions of the body or can slow down the metabolic process to make the body consume less energy,

From all these scientific observations, one can easily understand how Pranayama affects the various functions of the body. But the scientific work presented here is quite hazardous to extrapolate and say that the same would occur in every case.

The human body and its functions are always a matter of mystery. People having curious mind have tried to penetrate the fundamental difference between Pranayama Yoga and modern medicine with respect to basic sciences to justify that regular practice of Pranayama can eliminate mal functions of the body for perfect health and happiness.

Bibliography

1. The Essentials of Hinduism by: Swami Bhaskarananda
2. Ayurveda in classical Sanskrit Literature by: Anjalika Mukhaopadhyay
3. Yoga for women by:Nancy Phelan and Michael Volin
4. Yoga Simplified by: Shri Yogendra, 1959
5. Yoga Asanas simplified by: Shri Yogendra 1960
6. Yoga Self-Taught by: Andre Van Lysebeth
7. Raja yoga by: Swami Vivekananda
8. The synthesis of Yoga by: Sri Aurobindo, 1965
9. Extracts of Dr. Therese Brosse's phnemographic & cartographic recording.
10. Explanation of Prana, Swami Sivananda.
11. The spirit of Hinduism by: David Burnett. 1992.
12. Harmonic Gymnastic by: G. Stebbin. 1892 Edn,pp-771.
13. Essence of Pranayama by: Shirkrishna. 2012, Ishwardas chunilalyogic Health Centre.
14. 14. Integral healing: Compiled works of Sri Aurobindo and the Mother-2004
15. 15. Yoga Asanas simplified by Shri Yogendra, 1959
16. 16. Hinduism by: Swami Vivekananda -2004

Printed in the United States
by Baker & Taylor Publisher Services